The A Cappella Singer Who Lost Her Voice and Other Stories from NATURAL MEDICINE

By

Amy Rothenberg ND, DHANP

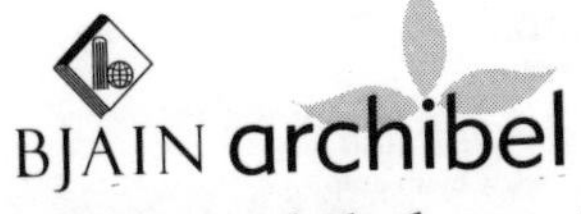

B. Jain Archibel s.p.r.l.

Rue Fontaine St. Pierre 1E, Zoning Industriel de la Fagne,

5330 Assesse, Belgium, Europe

THE A CAPPELLA SINGER WHO LOST HER VOICE AND OTHER STORIES FROM NATURAL MEDICINE

First Edition: 2011
1st Impression: 2011

Published by Kuldeep Jain for

B. JAIN ARCHIBEL S.P.R.L.
Rue Fontaine St. Pierre 1E, Zoning Industriel de la Fagne,
5330 Assesse, Belgium Europe
Tel.: +32 8266 55 00 • *Fax:* +32 83 65 62 82
Email: info@bjain.com • *Website:* **www.bjain.com**

B. JAIN PUBLISHERS (P) LTD.
An ISO 9001 : 2000 Certified Company
1921/10, Chuna Mandi, Paharganj, New Delhi 110 055 (INDIA)
Tel.: +91-11-4567 1000 • *Fax:* +91-11-4567 1010
Email: info@bjain.com • *Website:* **www.bjain.com**

Printed in India by
J.J. Offset Printers

ISBN: 978-2-87491-015-9

Disclaimer

Please be advised that though you may see yourself, a loved one or someone who resembles a patient of yours described in these pages, that treatment protocols in the world of natural medicine and in particular, in homeopathic prescribing, are above all, individualized. What works for one person will not necessarily work for another, even if there is a seemingly identical diagnosis. Please seek out the care or make a referral to a well thought of practitioner, especially if working with a patient who has a chronic illness. This work is not meant to replace that of a licensed physician or practitioner; please seek appropriate care.

Names and identifying information about patients have been changed to respect privacy; however, those described in this book are not composite images, but rather real patients with real lives.

Contents

Disclaimer .... *iii*

Acknowledgements .... *ix*

Preface .... *xv*

Chapters

1. Introduction.......... 1

- How I Landed in Naturopathic Medical School..........6
- Definitions and Descriptions of Naturopathic Medicine and Homeopathy..........10
- Who Visits a Naturopathic Doctor or a Homeopath?. 21
- A Typical Work Day..........23
- On Being a Teacher..........30
- On Working with One's Life Partner..........34

2. Introduction to Pregnancy and Small Children.......... 37

- Motherhood is the Mother of Invention! Babies, Babies, Babies..........37
- Infertility..........40
- Pregnancy..........43
- Ugliest Legs This Side of the Mississippi: A Case of Painful Varicose Veins in Pregnancy..........47

- Tips for New Moms and Families.....50
- Choosing Homeopathy for Children 53
- Wrap Up Those Babies!.....56
- Colic: The Curse of the Newborn.....58

3. For the Children in Your Life.....65

- Are You Giving Too Many Medicines to People in Your Family? Less is More! 65
- Homeopathy and Natural Medicine Help One Girl Step Up to the Plate!.....69
- Some Thoughts on Homeopathic Family Practice: Does Parenting Impact Constitutional Types? Should Constitutional Types in Children Impact Parenting? 73
- House Calls 83
- Special Children, Special Care.....85
- How to Stop the Fighting and Enhance Family Harmony.....97
- Mother's Day 108
- Asperger's Syndrome: Can Homeopathy Help?..... 111
- The Homeopathic Treatment of Autistic Spectrum Disorder 130

4. For Teenagers..... 135

- Teenagers, Gotta Love 'Em 135
- College Bound.....146
- Homeopathy from the Sidelines 153

5. For Adults..... 159

- Back to School Stress for Mom (Poison Ivy Story) ..159

- The Perfect Mother 163
- The A Cappella Singer Who Lost Her Voice 169
- Sneezing and Yelling: Two Parts of the Whole. Help with a Severe Case of Hay Fever 175
- 'Tis the Season to be Stressed Out, Fa-La-La-La-La: A Case of Chronic Sinusitis 180
- The Heart of the Matter: Homeopathy Helps with an Irregular Heartbeat 185
- The Man Who Married His Job: A Case of Chronic Heartburn and Acid Reflux 195
- Never Well Since the Flu 202
- From Nursing to Hot Flashes: A Middle-aged Mom's Dilemma 205
- Wear and Tear Arthritis: What Can Be Done to Ease the Pain? 211
- A Patient Story of Recurring Hives 215
- New Year's Resolutions: Increasing Energy and Resolve 223
- Stress Related Pain: A Case of Costochondritis 227
- Facing Cancer: What Can We Do? 232
- Meniere's: A Dizzying Disease 243
- When Muscles, Bones and Joints Go Out of Whack 253
- Irregular Paps, Genital Warts, Herpes 260

6. For Older Adults 269

- Getting Older, Getting Better 269
- The Lovely Man in the Fedora: A Case of Post-Herpetic Neuralgia 277

7. Special Topics 285

- Pharmaceuticals, Homeopathy and Natural Supplements: Can We Use All Together?..................285
- I Want to Be in the Olympics!......................................297
- In Conclusion...309

Acknowledgements

Without the many patients who have been under my care, there would be no book to write. I am appreciative of every person who ever came through my door and gave me the opportunity to offer care. And I am especially grateful to those who were patient with me as we tried to figure out the best approaches to healing. Patient stories at their root can be ordinary, extraordinary, complicated, heart wrenching or inspiring, or some combination thereof! The life stories my patients have shared in the context of our medical care relationships have kept my job interesting and challenging; it is to my patients I dedicate these pages.

To the many students and readers of my work, I am likewise indebted. You have driven my own study to understand what it is I do and gave me the opportunity to share it in ways that are informative, accessible, compelling and hopefully, at least sometimes, entertaining. If you can then take anything I share and use it help others, this is my greatest wish. Thank you for your confidence and trust in my lessons and in my words.

When I first met Kim McGuire, she had come to babysit for my three small children. She left with a bit of money in her pocket and a bad case of conjunctivitis! Thankfully, she agreed to come back in other roles, first to help out with office work related to publication of *The New England Journal of Homeopathy* and then the *Herscu Letter*. Kim is often the first person someone speaks to when inquiring about learning with the New England School of Homeopathy or with questions about our website. Kim has also worked the front office at my practice one day a week for many years. She brings an upbeat energy and dedication and accuracy to all she does as well as an empathetic posture to patients in my care. Kim truly understands many aspects of my work and is the best person I could hope to put forth to an inquiring public. Kim is quick to generate time saving and forward-thinking ideas for many aspects of my career. Her ability to stay gracious in the face of work-time overload is one of Kim's greatest strengths and I have grown to depend upon it.

Linda Smith has been my lead receptionist at the medical practice, keeping my paperwork in order and patient schedules in line. Linda has juggled many different kinds of patients with various needs and desires, often at the same time! Our waiting room is often circus-like and Linda does her best to remain affable. It's a job that requires patience and fortitude, which Linda continues to demonstrate, and I am indebted to her for being there week in, week out, dependable, organized and reliable. Between Linda and Kim nearly all administrative duties related to my work are handled, which frees me to focus my attention and thoughts to my patients, writing and teaching, as well as to the keeping of my home and the raising of my family.

Colleen Brophy arrived at our door; Mary Poppins-like, stayed four years when my children were small and literally saved my life! She is a second mother to my kids and allowed me to continue to have meaningful work outside the home, in addition to the important and challenging tasks of raising a family through the years of toddlerhood and preschool. I was also freed to exercise, have a social world and spend alone time with my husband and even travel a bit for work during that hectic time because Colleen was holding down the fort. The energy and creativity she brought into my life was no small gift. Now a mother of two herself, I owe her a dept of gratitude.

Mitzi Lebensorger, editor of *Homeopathy Today* (HT), has long been my editor and friend, since the early days of my teaching for the National Center for Homeopathy's summer school at Endicott College. We have developed a very harmonious working relationship: She gives me a deadline and I write her an article! Her clear understanding of homeopathy and her pitch perfect eye for what readers of HT want, has helped me to tailor and improve my writing for that particular audience. She captured the feeling and content of many of my pieces by entitling them and writing complementary sidebars; a number of her titles have crossed over into this book. I appreciate Mitzi's encouragement and her editorial support as well as her steadfast commitment to promoting and clarifying homeopathy for both the lay and professional reader.

Amy Mayer, a local writer on topics of health and education, was instrumental and encouraging to my launching this book. She also did early round editing on a number of the pieces in this volume. She was helpful at an important time for me and I appreciate her deep understanding of my profession, as well as her editorial eye. And thank you Amy for your ideas on a title for this book.

Liz Kaltman, MPH, ND came to study with us some years ago, with perhaps a modicum of trepidation. After completing our course on the east coast she moved her family to Oregon in order to pursue an ND degree. While there, she coordinated NESH classes and other teaching opportunities. Over the years, she has offered unending support for many aspects of my work and brings to it her own intelligence, bottomless energy and skillful organization. Most recently, she has contributed to our efforts in work related to public health.

The support of friends and extended family cannot be underestimated. Though I was slow to share this work with people, there were those always ready to urge me on to whom I am grateful: Lynn Bowmaster, Carole Horowitz, Cynthia Gensheimer, Robin Diamond, Ronni Blumenthal, Deb Habib, Tiina Booth, Jaymie Chernoff, Marina Goldman and Janet Monnier as well as my siblings, David, Joan and Nancy Rothenberg and Marla Brodsky. Also, knowing that I was writing for a long line of dedicated students and readers of my work, who have waited patiently for this book, kept my fingers at the keyboard even when other demands called.

My children, who drew so much out of me, have given back to me in spades. I could never have written this book without my experience of being a mother. Children can bring us to the very edge of sanity and overwhelm one minute and to tremendous love and pride the next. Building a family is filled with hard work, moments of grace, disappointment, exhilaration and just about everything in between. For every hour I put into caring for my children, loving them, cooking meals, reading stories, doing art projects, playing outside, going on trips far and wide, tending small illnesses and injuries, reading their writing, going camping, watching their friendships develop, cheering from the sidelines, worrying about this or that, talking with teachers, editing college essays; for every hour poured into those relationships, what I have now is the fact that they have grown into wonderful young adults. They are each full of passion, compassion, vision, intellect, the ability to work hard, have fun and perhaps most importantly, a deep capacity for love. With all the troubles of the world, I know at the very least, I am leaving behind three people, who with their dreams and aspirations, their talent and work ethic, will help make the world a better place.

SO, in *alphabetical* order:

Jonah, last to arrive, but first one ready to go, unflappable in most every way, models for our family patience, calmness and the benefits of consistent, indefatigable positive thinking. If you were ever to doubt yourself, Jonah would be right there to shore you up. He has always had the uncanny ability to bring all kinds of people readily into his circle with his easy-going nature and natural kindness. His hard work, athletic prowess, self-determination and gregarious temperament are the gifts he brings to this world and inspire me.

Misha I can look to for motivation in his prevailing thirst for knowledge and his flawless self-discipline. His curiosity informs his posture in the world and his ability to see connections across and between seemingly disparate disciplines. A dreamer with his feet on the ground, Misha feels deeply, experiences life with both an open heart *and* a discriminating eye. He is a devoted friend, a natural scholar and accomplished athlete. I am forced to keep learning and to work harder from Misha.

Sophie, my firstborn, has always been the queen of empathy and knowing perceptiveness about people. Her exuberance and ability to read people and situations is fine-tuned and she articulates her perceptions and feelings with nuanced understanding. Her strong mind and the unbridled joy she shares from her worlds of academics, performance and competitive athletics scoops people into her ever-widening and overlapping circles; her strength of vision, her steadfast dedication to everything she holds dear, stirs in me the same desire.

My children's support of my work is an ongoing blessing. This book is for you kids, may you each go from strength to strength, and always know Papa and I love you, we believe in you, we're there for you, and of course: there's no problem so big you can't solve!

To my parents, who died when I was quite young, I am grateful for their love and affection.

We all know that behind every visionary man there is the woman. In many of the settings of my family's life and my husband's work, that would be me! What may be less apparent is that my husband, Paul Herscu ND, has also stood behind me with unwavering adoration and endless encouragement. It does not matter what I want to do or do not want to do, Paul supports my process, my decisions and my choices; he further applauds my efforts and relishes in my accomplishments large and small. I am the most fortunate person in the world to have found a partner I can love and admire, enjoy and embrace and whom I continue to find both adorable and brilliant. There is more on Paul elsewhere in this book, as it is around him that I have built and will continue to build my life.

Preface

I devoured my earliest Oliver Sachs book when I was nursing my first child. I was captured by his eloquent descriptions of patients, their lives, their illnesses and his unique experiences of and with them. Sachs brought patients to life and provided my first exposure to narrative medicine. I appreciated the way he shared his own feelings and emotions *vis-a-vis* his patients. In a brazen move, fueled by enthusiasm and a strongly affiliative nature, I sent Dr. Sachs a copy of a journal I was working on at the time; it was a neurology issue of the *New England Journal of Homeopathy*. I sent it because I felt a kinship, an affinity; because I, too, met with patients for long initial visits and took time to understand their lives. I worked with people over years and decades. Due to the nature of my work, I, too, necessarily had to understand my patients' pathologies in the context of their life experiences. And I have been similarly engulfed and moved by many of my patients' stories. Though I hope and believe I have helped many of those I have treated, it is certain that they have helped me. They helped me to grow into a more compassionate and patient doctor, drove my understanding of humanity, facilitated my ability to see and experience the breath and depth of suffering that individuals endure, and offered me insight into the inspirational resilience of the human body and spirit.

In this book, I aim to do the same for you. My field, naturopathic medicine, is the state-of-the-art complementary and alternative medicine field burgeoning at the beginning of this millenium. Under this licensure, I practiced exceedingly full time for some years and consistently part time for many. Alongside therapeutic nutrition, botanical medicine and lifestyle recommendations, I utilize homeopathy with most every patient. In homeopathy I have found a definitively holistic approach where each patient is understood in terms of their physical, psychological, emotional and cognitive states, where the imbalance or discomfort or disease is relevant alongside the whole person and their story. How a patient fits into the environment where they live, work and play becomes as important as how they are influenced by, and in turn influence their surroundings. I try to understand symptoms as an expression of a predictable and patterned way a particular patient responds to stressors in their life. Learning to use the tool of homeopathy, which is alternately quite simple and then immensely complicated, is a lifelong pursuit.

The cases and stories in this book present a wide breath of patient experiences. You will ascertain the strong and underlying philosophy that informs my work. You will start to see what kinds of things are important to this practitioner of natural medicine. You can start to understand the sorts of results, in term of symptoms, in terms of lab work, in terms of pace of healing that are part of what I do. You will see that not everyone can be helped, that alongside celebrated successes, like most every doctor, I have some stunning failures. It is those people that do not get well, who keep me up at night and keep me learning, trying to understand new applications or new approaches, that I might better assist a suffering person.

I hope what emerges is a greater understanding of how I practice as well as an appreciation of the gentle effectiveness and power of natural medicine. Many patients are looking to complementary and alternative approaches for both prevention and treatment of all manner of illness. There are many answers and many paths to healing. This path is the one that I offer and in it have found meaningful, challenging and inspiring work. I am rarely bored and never complacent. There is always more to learn, more people and families to try to help and support.

I have spent more than two decades immersed in clinical work and also in teaching and writing for lay and physician audiences. Knowing that I may be writing or teaching about a particular illness, natural remedy or clinical skill sharpens my own proficiency, especially during my time with patients. I want to be as accurate and forthcoming as possible. I strive to break things down to component parts, to be transparent in my work and my writing, so that nothing is hidden and there are no tricks unshared. We sometimes hear the adage, *those who can, do, those who can't, teach.* Though that might be true for some, I hope in my case my capacity for and joy derived from writing and teaching remains fueled by an intense desire to let others authentically in on what I do. Like most who do something for a long time, it naturally, even necessarily, becomes second nature. But to teach a beginner how to take a thorough case history or to motivate someone who is feeling stuck professionally to improve their technique, I hear as a calling. I do it with an openness and accessibility. No one can teach someone how to be a doctor, but by modeling what I do and by trying to explain all the details, I can at very least present one way to work. And if I am doing my job well, I am rousing others to find what it is they can bring to their field, to their patients, to the healing of the sick.

Additionally, to put forward this information spreads the word about complementary and alternative medicine (CAM), its elegance and efficacy, its promise and potential. I have not aimed to be comprehensive in this volume, nor is it a 'how to' book. Rather, I am offering a serious glimpse into the life of a naturopathic physician, both in and out of the office. I began as an educated, ardent doctor, newly married, without children, in the plains of Nebraska and landed some years later in the idyllic and stimulating life of Amherst, Massachusetts where I have put down roots and raised a family. My home life and in particular, being a mother, has enlightened my work as a physician. My career as a doctor has profoundly influenced my home life and relationships. In many ways having part-time, meaningful and well-paying work outside the home during the early years of raising a family was a kind of lifeline that in fact, inspired my life as a homemaker.

If I can create a kind of world for you to enter, for information or diversion, clinical pearls or understanding, I am happy to do so. If this book encourages you or someone you know to consider a career in medicine or CAM or encourages you or a loved one to seek out medical care, my work is, at least for the time being, done. And that is not something most women can say!

Amy Rothenberg, ND
Amherst, Massachusetts
Mother's Day 2010

Chapter 1

Introduction

Some of the chapters in this book are adapted from articles written for *Homeopathy Today* (HT), the publication of the National Center for Homeopathy. There I worked with the late, indomitable Julian Winston, who was the longtime editor of HT and afterward and more consistently with Mitzi Lebensorger. Julian was happy to have any copy to work with and encouraged me to write whatever I felt like writing. He was entertaining, discriminating, persnickety and I miss him dearly. Mitzi was often looking for specific pieces but was also open to what I was thinking about at any given time. Mitzi's understanding of homeopathy along with her layperson's sensibility helped me craft pieces that were accessible, informative *and* I hope, enjoyable to read; I owe her a great debt.

My aim has always been to write so people could learn, to share honestly from my experience as a physician, and to leave readers with some new element of understanding or something to think about. The focus of many of these pieces has been homeopathy, but I would often also offer my thoughts about other natural medicine modalities to the pathology discussed or for the patient at hand as that best reflected my work in the clinic.

What these chapters describe is my evolution over time as a naturopathic physician specializing in classical homeopathy. I utilize a range of modalities in order to help my patients. I also work with patients to help reduce and manage stress in their lives and I encourage exercise or movement as a key component to health. Likewise eating healthful, balanced and appropriate diets, and remembering to rest enough may often become part of a treatment plan. I seem to increasingly spend time with patients helping them strategize about ways to create more harmonious workplaces and to troubleshoot problems and issues at home related to partners, children, friends and parents.

My training as a naturopathic physician had girded me with a whole array of options to share with my patients and that is what I have always done. Beyond helping patients at the moment of their visits, I am also invested in teaching and modeling for them prevention techniques and general healthy living. The goal, after all, is not just to have patients be symptom-free or to minimize complaints but also to lead patients toward more robust energy as well as mental clarity and emotional freedom so they can do what they need to do and also pursue things in life they love.

Most of the pieces in this collection were written over the ten year period of 1998-2008. During that time my growth as a physician continued and my responsibilities as a teacher grew. Many of these writings though not all, have been previously published in journals and magazines or have been used as teaching tools in academic settings. I have received letters, calls and emails from readers afar thanking me for writing and wishing they could find similar material to read. It is my hope that in this volume, practitioners, at-home prescribers and others interested in the elegant and gentle ways of natural medicine and homeopathy in particular, will find useful and inspiring reading. It is my dream that all who find their way to natural medicine also find their way to help further its reach, through the sharing of stories, the discussion of ideas and the word of mouth communication that happens when we are enthusiastic about any subject matter.

In this time of tremendous medical advances, we also find many people still suffering, suffering in the physical realm and also struggling psychologically and spiritually. A deep acting medicine, such as homeopathy, aims to bring balance and ease into patients' lives and at its best, does just that. Even at times of great distress and worry, we can hope to ease symptoms and renew balance. Natural medicine does not offer a panacea for every condition or for every person, but when used by well-trained providers it aims to address the deeper imbalances that cause pathology and works to help patients discover healthier ways to approach their healthcare.

In my experience as a student, practitioner and teacher my best learning has happened primarily in the clinical setting and secondly, through reading accounts of patients. I hope that by reading through these pages, you might find the common threads, the themes that underlie the way one practitioner sees the world and how I use CAM right alongside other medical and healing modalities. In terms of homeopathy specifically, you will begin to appreciate the kind of information that is of interest and relevance to the homeopath.

These articles can be read sequentially, one at a time or in any order. I have grouped them by the patient stage of life as one way to organize the body of work. That said, I am always looking at the whole person in front of me at the time of any visit. I am trying to understand their pathology or illness in the context of the rest of their lives at that point in time. So, such distinctions are not essential. Feel free to read this book back to front or every other section if you prefer; the chapters should have a cumulative effect in whatever order they are examined.

I have recorded a CD which answers most every question new patients have asked me. In my practice, I actually collected those questions over a two-year period of time and then set out to thoughtfully answer each one. The first few minutes of that CD can also be found as a podcast on the website www.nesh.com if you would like to share that bit with others. You can also order the CD from the web address.

A note of precaution. Natural medicine, above all, is medicine that is individualized to the patient. If you read about a patient in these pages who has a similar diagnosis to you, a loved one or a patient of yours, do not assume that they will respond similarly to the same treatment plan or protocol or homeopathic remedy. If I have eight patients with arthritis, they might be prescribed eight different remedies or perhaps six different homeopathic remedies, varying dietary recommendations and perhaps nutritional supplements particular to their unique presentation. Always I am basing my prescriptions on how the patients experience their pathology and also how that illness fits into the rest of their overall health, as well as other elements of their lives.

In homeopathy we call this *constitutional prescribing* and find it to be a most effective and deep-acting way to use homeopathy. We give the best-matched remedy at the lowest possible strength to help the patient. You can find some homeopaths that will offer remedies in a more cookbook fashion based on the name of the disease. But, in my mind and in my hand, I have found constitutional homeopathic prescribing to hold the most potential for healing the sick and preventing disease.

Likewise, in the larger world of CAM, individualizing treatment plans is one of the most important elements of practice. I share in these pages many of the other CAM approaches that I use alongside homeopathy in my practice. Trained in naturopathic medicine, I often think broadly. Most every patient I see, I do use homeopathy; but therapeutic nutrition, botanical medicine, home remedies and lifestyle recommendations are also commonly part of my patient protocols. Through patient education and encouragement, I am able to empower patients and parents of patients to take better care of themselves and their families with an eye toward prevention, as well as the treatment of common ailments.

In the context of my work I also often have the need to refer to other healthcare providers for both diagnostic and treatment support. I am lucky to live in an area where there are many open-minded doctors and have a well-established referral network. And those referrals go both ways. There are frequently patients for whom the orthodox medical world cannot offer much. Perhaps the problem itself is incurable, or perhaps the pharmaceutical approach is not working, not working well enough, or causing intolerable side effects. I do my best with the patients sent to me by others and sometimes, even if I cannot help with the particular chief complaint, I may well be able to help with the mind set, the sleep, digestion, etc. And because I have a medical training, I can communicate effectively with medical colleagues and share resources and experiences.

I had the honor of serving for six years on the town of Amherst, Massachusetts' Board of Health beginning in the late 90's. One of the most satisfying accomplishments of that tenure was passing a ruling, which banned smoking in bars in this small New England college town. We met quite a bit of resistance, most especially from bar owners and in general, from local citizens who did not want change. But now some years later, the economic impact of the ban is non-existent, the health of those working in bars is improved and all the people of this area can enjoy a smoke free environment in all indoor places. I bring up this story as a reflection of a paradigm shift that we are in the midst of, which also includes a shift towards medicine that is gentle, natural and effective and which can be used side by side other medical approaches. Interested people, patients and healthcare providers, alike, are now seeking after what was once met with resistance and trepidation.

How I Landed in Naturopathic Medical School

A few months after my twelfth birthday I was awakened suddenly in the early hours before dawn by ambulance lights swirling around the bedroom walls I shared with my sister. I heard banging around in the hallway outside my door and loud unfamiliar voices. I woke from that deep sleep to learn that my father had died.

Right there in his bedroom next to my own, with my mother at his side, my father lay, no longer in this world. The black mark the gurney made on our narrow hallway doorjamb stayed for months, a painful reminder of that auspicious summer morning. He, like many through the middle part of the twentieth century, was a two-pack-a day smoker, had stressful work and a family to support. With elevated blood pressure, high cholesterol and being overweight, the massive heart attack that killed him that quiet summer dawn, at least in hindsight, was no surprise. In those days, his only prescription was high blood pressure medication. Period. No weight loss recommendation, no stress reduction techniques, no encouragement for exercise, no dietary suggestions, no fish oil supplements or CoQ10.

We had a week of mourning in community where loved ones would come to the house. Invariably people showed up with ice cream, no party in July would be complete for Harry without ice cream. Our freezer was filled to capacity for months. After some time, our family life somehow came back to some semblance of normal. There is a way that the daily routines of school and socializing and 4-H club meetings and sports brought a sense of the ordinary back to me. As an engaged junior high school student, I was likely living in a somewhat oblivious adolescent bubble.

But loss was not to be a one time knock at our family's door. A brief time later, my mother was diagnosed with breast cancer to which she succumbed some four years after my father. Perhaps the stress and grief of losing a great love, not to mention the father to her children and the main breadwinner, proved too great a stress for my mother. She, too, was a heavy smoker and did not have healthy living habits, though she did seem to be in fine health before her diagnosis.

As a sixteen year old, now without parents, the fact that the medical treatments of the time offered virtually nothing to my own parents, soured my childhood aspiration of becoming a doctor. I figured, if there was so little help available for people with such common and major illness in general, and to my family in particular, it would be best to find some sort of profession that would be more satisfying, more fulfilling.

Despite that most unusual adolescence and being somewhat unguided, I did surprisingly well in school. My high school guidance counselor, Ferne Goldstein, was quite certain I would do best in a college where learning *how* to think and being creative would be emphasized. She imagined that I would do well in a place that required work and that internships, the practical part of learning, would appeal to me. Four days after my high school graduation, I left for Antioch College in Yellow Springs, Ohio, to begin in the summer session, brimming with ideas of what I would like to study: journalism, poetry, philosophy, art. The environment there suited me well, smart students and original thinkers, creative spirits living collectively in a pristine and wild place. I thrived.

And though I consciously tried to embrace the humanities, at every turn, I was pulled into the wide world of science, especially biology, biochemistry, botany and nutrition. It seemed my natural interests ran deep and instinctively in those directions; I was able to grasp the material and integrate information with ease. I was commonly on the verge of utter exhilaration over learning new things and though I also enjoyed my humanities and social science classes, they paled next to my unbridled enthusiasm for the natural world.

I remember fondly my academic advisor, the late Jim Howell, aptly named for an ornithologist, who, with his beak-like nose and black-rimmed classes and diminutive stature looked every bit a small eager bird. He consistently fed my enthusiasm for the sciences and applauded each of my academic accomplishments. He also unearthed my long held, yet buried interest in medicine and started a small flame of desire in that direction, though I proved resistant.

As part of my undergraduate work, I had the tremendous opportunity for an internship at a research lab at the Oregon Health Sciences University in Portland. I am slightly embarrassed to say that I hitchhiked there from Ohio and landed in downtown Portland. My first stop was a health food store to find something to eat. Browsing the bulletin board I saw this sign: 'Three Naturopathic Students Looking for a Housemate.' Having never seen the word 'naturopathic,' I honestly thought it pertained to people who worked in trail maintenance or the like! But, it was a good location and the price was right. The other housemates seemed to like me well enough, so later that week, I moved in.

Well! *These people were doing exactly what I wanted to do.* They were passionate about their class work and overflowing with stories from their clinical experiences. They were immersed in the hard sciences but also open to the more subtle elements of healing. They talked about developing relationships with patients that were meaningful and mutually satisfying. They were concerned with research in natural medicine while curious about folk medicine and the healing work done by practitioners in the developing world. They were committed to living healthfully and spreading the word and work of natural and holistic healing.

I believe that there was more than a smidgeon of divine intervention that led me to that southeast Portland bungalow and into the lives of these capable and inspired naturopathic medical school students. To find a career built to the dimensions I had dreamed of, exactly the kind of medical work I could relate to, I knew I "had arrived." At the young age of 20, I left Oregon and heading back to Yellow Springs to finish my prerequisites to apply to the National College of Naturopathic Medicine (NCNM). I graduated with a degree in biology in June and began NCNM that August.

This time, I *drove* to Oregon with a friend, with all my worldly possessions packed into two large boxes. No parents to set me on this course, no partner to consult, no one I knew who had taken this path, or even heard of it for that matter, but with a strong unwavering belief that I had what it would take to get through the training and be prepared to offer a gentle, natural and effective approach to the prevention and treatment of illness. If there is such a thing as destiny, surely it was driving the hand of those advising me those early years and supporting me along the way.

Definitions and Descriptions of Naturopathic Medicine and Homeopathy

Before you begin this book it will be helpful to know some basic background and terminology about this profession. As a naturopathic physician, I attended a four year, in-residence naturopathic medical school. The first two years of that program cover the basic sciences, much like a more typical medical school. We spend the first year learning about the human body in "normal" state by studying among other things, anatomy, physiology and biochemistry. We work on cadavers to get a first hand experience of the human body looks like, inside and out.

In the second year we learn how everything can go wrong. We study physical and clinical diagnosis learning how to perform a complete physical examination; we study laboratory diagnosis, X-ray diagnosis and pathology along with learning how to interpret findings. We also begin in these first two years learning about naturopathic medical philosophy and history. Between the first two years, we begin to see patients in the outpatient clinics under the supervision of licensed physicians. The third and fourth year are devoted to the systems review classes such as EENT, Gastroenterology, Dermatology, Gynecology, Cardiology, Urology, etc., as well as the natural medicine modalities that are the hallmark of this profession: therapeutic nutrition through diet and supplements, nature cure approaches that include hydrotherapy and fasting, botanical medicine, using tinctures, extracts, poultices and other preparations, Chinese medicine, physical medicine which includes naturopathic manipulation and massage, and homeopathy.

Many students choose to specialize in one area of the body or in one or another therapeutic modality. For instance, a naturopathic physician may choose to specialize in Sports Medicine or in Cardiology. Others may decide to focus on Chinese medicine or therapeutic nutrition. For each of these specialties there is generally additional training, both in the classroom and the clinic as well as further credentialing requirements. In all, over 2000 hours must be logged in seeing patients in the clinic, practicing the skills in terms of physical exams as well as case taking, patient relationship and actual analysis of the situation after which a medical plan, with follow up recommendation, is created with the guidance of more experienced and legally responsible licensed physicians.

Naturopathic physicians are licensed as primary care providers, at this time, in 13 states. There are also currently 22 states in legislative efforts. We have long believed there is no stopping an idea whose time has come and the American people are clamoring for physician level practitioners of natural medicine. Every state that licenses NDs also requires proof of continuing education coursework as well as malpractice insurance. Many NDs work in the private practice settings, some in group practices and others in hospital or integrative care centers. Others teach, write or conduct research; many do a combination of the above.

I chose toward the end of my education to specialize in homeopathy. Homeopathy is a unique system of medicine which addresses the whole patient - physically, mentally and emotionally. Symptoms are understood according to the classic physiologic model taught to all health care providers. As the patient strains against both internal and external stressors the patient develops symptoms; the symptoms are seen as the person's way of handling this dynamic. It is the gleaning and understanding of the details of and connections among these symptoms that lead the homeopath to prescribe a particular remedy.

Homeopathy was first conceived by Samuel Hahnemann (1755-1843), a German physician and chemist. Troubled by the harshness of medical protocols of his time as well as by personal family tragedies, he turned away from medical practice and devoted himself to the work of scientific translation. It was during his work on a translation of a popular book on botanical medicine, Cullen's *Materia Medica* from the English into German. He became intrigued with the portion written on Cinchona bark, from which quinine was eventually derived and the close relationship between its effectiveness and its toxicity. His curiosity was ignited.

He undertook what were essentially the first drug trials, known as *provings*—giving healthy subjects samples of the substance in question and seeing what, if any, effect it had upon them. To his surprise, in the case of the Cinchona bark, a number of participants developed the very symptoms that the herbal preparation was known to help.

From this observation was born *similia similibus curantur* from the Latin, "likes are cured by likes." This essential underpinning of homeopathic practice can be further defined as follows: Any drug which is capable of producing morbid symptoms in the healthy will remove similar symptoms occurring as an expression of disease. In his lifetime, Hahnemann conducted provings on some 106 substances. He worked diligently and wrote prolifically on topics of homeopathic philosophy, the treatment of chronic disease as well as the *Materia Medica Pura,* one of the earliest homeopathic drug compendiums available.

Hahnemann also set out to determine what the optimal dosage of medication would be to achieve both best clinical outcomes and the least side effects. His ideas about using the minimal dose whenever possible have stood the test of time. His experimentations led to concepts of dilution and succussion, which are used in the potentization process of the homeopathic remedies. At this time, homeopathic remedies are made in accordance to the United States Homeopathic Pharmacopoeia and are produced from plant, mineral and animal sources. Homeopathic remedies are available through homeopathic pharmacies as well as over-the-counter in some pharmacies and health food stores.

Homeopathy is used to treat first aid problems as well as acute and chronic disease. First aid problems are addressed in a rather 'cookbook' fashion. For example, many have heard of using the homeopathic remedy *Arnica montana* for the treatment of trauma. Because traumatic events impact most people in a similar fashion, *Arnica* is one of only a handful of remedies to be considered. In other words, when the stress from the outside is very severe, most individuals respond in a similar fashion. That response will point to one of only a few remedies.

For acute, self-limited problems such as otitis media, cystitis or diarrhea, patients present in a more individualized manner. For instance, one person with diarrhea might have copious flatulence, stomachache and feel chilly while another might feel warm, and simultaneously have a pounding headache. Though both have diarrhea, they would require and respond to two different homeopathic remedies. The homeopath is addressing the whole person at any one time. With most acute illness there are a limited number of remedies to choose from because there are only so many ways an acute problem can manifest.

When patients present in the office with what *appears* to be an acute problem, we are interested to understand if it is *truly an acute problem* or if it is rather a flare up of an underlying chronic condition. This would be true in illnesses for which flare-ups are common such as multiple sclerosis, migraine headache and premenstrual syndrome, but can also be found in those with upper respiratory tract infection, sinusitis, cystitis, or digestive complaints, etc. Differentiating at this juncture informs treatment options and impacts both the homeopathic remedy choice and dosage.

For illnesses which are more chronic in nature, homeopathic practitioners prescribe *constitutional* remedies, which are based on the whole person, including symptoms of the chief complaint(s). Homeopathic remedies are given for particular people, as opposed to particular diagnoses. One could have five patients with chronic migraine headache and they might receive five different remedies depending on how they experience the problem; that is, how it actually feels, the type of pain or discomfort, what makes it better, what makes it worse, is there a clear initial etiology, does anything bring on each episode, do they have any other symptoms simultaneously, etc. The homeopath is interested in how the headache fits into the rest of the person's physical health. In addition, it is central to perceive how those physical characteristics sit *vis a' vis* the patients' mental and emotional health.

To the homeopath, all symptoms are *context dependent*; one cannot see a symptom standing by itself, rather the homeopath seeks to understand each symptom a patient reports as it relates to the whole person. The typical intake for a homeopathic physician is one and half to two hours, allowing enough time to fully understand the patient and all aspects of their lifestyle and health. Thus, the doctor-patient relationship is an important component of the homeopathic process.

Our individualized approach would be utilized regardless of the main complaint. For some patients, there are very few outward symptoms related to their pathology making it seemingly difficult for the homeopath to prescribe upon such a chief complaint. However, the homeopath can prescribe based on *presenting symptoms from all systems of the body* and from general physical characteristics of the patient as well as from their mental and emotional make-up. Homeopathic physicians give a remedy for the patient and expect their overall health to improve, including presenting symptoms. Often there is clear pathology and the patient reports clear symptomatology. The homeopath analyzes this information, seeking to understand it in context of the whole patient.

There are no charts to turn to or PDRs to reference offering linear, specific recommendations and dosages, but that does not mean there are no tools of the trade. Homeopaths study this medical art by focusing on a number of subjects. There is the ongoing study of *materia medica* - learning each remedy and how patients who need it would present with regard to all physical symptoms, that is, in a review of systems fashion. Homeopaths learn how each constitutional remedy type would present with regard to the mental and emotional characteristics as well. The study of *materia medica* is a life long pursuit. Differential *materia medica,* in which remedies that are similar to each other are studied together furthers helps the prescriber when it comes time to make the appropriate prescription. Authors are known based on their style of prose or on their practical experience. The rich literature of this profession was recently highlighted in a book by Julian Winston entitled, *The Heritage of Homeopathic Literature–An Abbreviated Bibliography and Commentary*, which is worth a perusal by anyone interested in either the history of writing which has accompanied and grown this medical approach or the practical, well-referenced overview this volume offers.

The practice of homeopathy includes on-going study of case-analysis techniques with a focus on the long-term follow-up of patients. The goal is to be able to treat a patient through their lives, through the acute and chronic illnesses that may arise. Assessing efficacy and deciding the course of treatment requires a strong philosophical understanding of the homeopathic healing process and the nature of the person and their pathology. It is not uncommon to revisit the homeopathic philosophy books, particularly when faced with a complicated patient.

To help facilitate recall of these some 2000 remedies in use, many homeopaths study and then refer to repertories, which are books which list all the symptoms known and the homeopathic remedies which have helped treat those specific symptoms. Repertories are organized by parts of the body. The mind section, so essential in our assessment, is followed by the head, eyes, ears, nose, face, mouth, teeth, throat, stomach, abdomen, rectum, stool, bladder, kidneys, prostate, urethra, urine, male genitalia, female genitalia, larynx and trachea, respiration, cough, chest, back, extremities, sleep, dreams, chill, fever, perspiration, skin and generalities. In this age of computer technology, these volumes are now available by computer program.

"Repertorization" of a patient's case can be done in a timely fashion after a full homeopathic interview, helping guide the homeopathic physician to a group of the most likely remedies to be considered for a particular patient. One still needs to perceive the correct symptomatology and to understand the patient in all aspects of their health, as even the best computer program would be of little use if the incorrect information was considered. Then, the prescribing homeopath must choose the correct remedy from a group of those suggested. Computers have made this work of analysis less cumbersome and certainly less time-consuming. Additionally, computer technology allows the qualified homeopath to be flexible with regard to various analysis techniques.

It should also be added, that homeopaths prescribe just as often by pattern recognition. After one has treated fifteen or twenty patients who responded well to the remedy *Nux vomica*, for instance, it is not difficult to recognize that pattern in the next patient who presents and needs the remedy. So, even though a complete case is taken, by the end of the office visit the homeopath would ask questions which are geared at *confirming* a particular remedy and ruling out others. Like any physician, some prescriptions are routine and others require much study, perhaps a conversation with colleagues or research of the literature.

Another field of study and reference volumes homeopaths peruse are those on the topic of therapeutics or homeopathic remedy protocols based on systems of the body. This focus is somewhat inconsistent with the understanding in homeopathy–that the prescriptions be based on the person, not the diagnosis. Yet some remedies have an affinity for certain kinds of problems which tend to arise in certain types of people. The remedies can therefore be grouped and studied in such a fashion via comparative *materia medica* offering the prescribing homeopath the ability to more easily differentiate between similar remedies as well as similar patients.

Like other physicians and healers we study cured cases which are published in peer-reviewed homeopathic journals to better understand the impact of the remedies on actual patients as well as to keep abreast on new findings within the profession.

Similar to all areas of medicine, some patients are eager to self-prescribe. There are many resources available to the layperson interested in homeopathy, from books and magazines, to websites and computer programs. It is hoped that most self-prescribers or those who dabble with their family's first aid and acute healthcare problems understand the need for professional assistance when a problem is severe, long lasting or complicated. This issue is not limited to those who use homeopathic remedies at home, but could be said for all who opt out of the use of medical expertise: The biggest dangers lie in missed diagnoses and the loss of valuable time in addressing treatable conditions. Natural medicines in general have lower toxicity and cause fewer side effects than many allopathic medications, but nothing is perfectly safe.

Like other medications there are recommended dosages. The strength, quantity and frequency of the prescription are individualized to the patient as much as the remedy itself. Things that are taken into consideration when the dosage is made include: the patient's age and size, type and severity of pathology and other medications currently being taken.

Most homeopathic remedies are applied to small lactose pellets and taste sweet. The pellets are taken, allowed to dissolve under the tongue, away from food and drink. It is safe to give these small pellets to infants and those with difficulty swallowing. Remedies can also be dissolved in water and administered that way.

Some patients may present having self-prescribed combination remedies, which are available over the counter at health food stores and some pharmacies. These products have not undergone the accepted drug research protocols (provings) that *single homeopathic remedies* have, and are not applied in a manner consistent with homeopathic theory. It is possible that the patient needs one of the remedies included in the combination remedy and it will therefore have some effect, but it is generally not a profound or long-lasting one. Likewise, recently there have appeared homeopathic combination patch remedies which would raise the same concerns.

There have been numerous studies on homeopathy which have appeared in the orthodox medical literature. Notably, the *Lancet* published a review article in 1997 which was a meta-analysis of 89 blinded, randomized, placebo-controlled clinical trials. The trials looked at homeopathic treatment of such complaints as hay fever, asthma, rheumatoid arthritis, diarrhea, influenza, varicose veins, strains and sprains, and post-surgical complications. Patients who received homeopathic medications were 2.45 times more likely to receive a positive response than those given placebo which should encourage further and more widespread clinical and laboratory study of the efficacy and mechanism of action of homeopathic remedies. Many studies done have suffered from poor study design and there is movement in the integrative medicine world to correct those errors. Most all practitioners as well as the insurance industry, agree that better and more consistent studies would not only be welcome, but are essential to the growth of all aspects of integrative medicine.

I have found in homeopathy an approach to healing that is period intrinsically holistic. I always needed to understand the whole person, to understand the context of their symptoms and to see the illnesses as that person's way of responding to various known and unknown stressors. I liked that remedies could be given for one seemingly clear complaint and the patient would come back claiming other things had also improved. A gentle and curious modality, homeopathy struck my fancy. But not only that, I saw and continue to see, day in and day out in the clinic, that it is both safe and effective. And the process used to help decide which remedy to give to which patient for which kind of complaint, suits my ability in getting to know people and my natural curiosity about patient's lives. Perhaps homeopathy is not intuitively understandable to all, but hopefully the patients described in this book and their experiences with homeopathy will illustrate the ideas and realities behind this medicine, as well as how homeopathy can be utilized in the context of a broader approach to complementary medicine.

Who Visits A Naturopathic Doctor or a Homeopath?

Most practitioners of naturopathic medicine or homeopathy see a wide range of patients similar to that which a family doctor would encounter. Perhaps nothing else is working for a particular patient. For some known and some unknown reasons, there are patients who do not respond well to medications, some have paradoxical reactions to drugs, some are allergic to pharmaceuticals or do not tolerate them well.

Some patients merely want their medicine to be in accord with an overall health-oriented, natural lifestyle.

Some patients come to us because they have incurable conditions and are strictly seeking symptomatic or palliative care. Others seek to enhance immune function thereby reducing susceptibility to acute illness from which they suffer along with chronic complaints. Patients also make appointments in order to help address underlying mental, emotional or cognitive concerns which accompany chronic physical complaints.

The last group of people we may see are patients who do not feel well, yet there is nothing diagnostically wrong. Lab work, physical exam and health history are unremarkable, yet their vitality is diminished, there are low grade symptoms on various systems and the mood is depressed. Some of these patients have clear and intense subjective symptoms, but they continue to pass all exams. One of the unique benefits of complementary medical care is that since we treat the whole patient and we are concerned with how the whole system operates, we do not have to wait until the person presents with full-blown symptomatology. With regard to homeopathy in particular, the fact that there are not specific homeopathic remedies for specific diagnoses may make some uncomfortable; it is contrary to the modern medical model where drug prescriptions are most often diagnosis-driven. But, if there is no clear pathologic diagnosis, it can become difficult to choose correct medications or sometimes to provide any treatment at all. This is an added advantage of naturopathic medicine and homeopathic care: As a method of primary prevention, it can offer preventive approaches to patients *before* they become severely ill.

A Typical Work Day

My inner alarm clock goes off at 6:00 a.m. on the dot. I yank myself from the comfort of my bed and warmth of my sleeping husband. There is much to do this school-day morning. Over breakfast, the kids talk about the day before them, how prepared they are for their classes and what's happening after school. While I'm busy at the kitchen counter making sandwiches, I absorb the kids' slumber-filled quiet. As I wait for the toast to pop, I do some dishes and begin to shift modes. Once the kids are out the door, I tidy up the kitchen, throw in a load of laundry, check my email and start to think about the workday ahead of me.

On the road by 7:45, I head to the office where I have practiced naturopathic medicine since my mid twenties. The Connecticut River Valley offers sweeping views of the Holyoke Mountains as I make my way over a notch in this range that runs, unlike most mountain ranges, from east to west. This is Mt. Norwottock that I see from the bay window of my kitchen, making up one side of the container that creates the Pioneer Valley. I slip though sleepy South Hadley with Mt. Holyoke College sitting importantly in her grey stone walled buildings and manicured grounds. I can pick up the highway right outside of town and be to work in a half hour. When my children were younger, I disliked the commute; I felt it took precious time away from my family, but now, I relish the quiet alone time in the car, a chance to totally change gears and prepare myself for a day in the clinic.

I will see patients, talk to perspective patients on the phone and address paper work that goes along with the job. I will work for seven or eight hours, without many breaks. I will hopefully help most who come my way; I will refer some for further diagnostic or laboratory work or to other practitioners. I will interact with patients and parents of patients by telephone, fax, letter and email, fielding questions about symptoms and protocols. The day will move quickly, with happy tales, heartbreaking stories and plenty of information for me to process. I will need to be alert and compassionate, calling on hard-earned knowledge from many years of study and over two decades of practice. If it is like most work days for me, I will leave knowing how blessed I am to have a job filled with intellectual challenges, satisfying interpersonal interactions and the awareness that I am having a positive impact on people's lives.

When I first began practice, like many of my naturopathic physician colleagues, I was zealous. I felt there was no one I could not assist and no patient pathology that I would not welcome the chance to try to understand and help. When I began this work there were harried days packed with patients, never time for lunch and much to be done in the library after hours. There was a kind of insanity that went along with the first years of practice, a time of total immersion and surrender to the work.

Paul, who I have practiced with since the get go, and I would have lunch in the back room, wolfing down sandwiches between patients and snacking on nuts and raisins. We were not practicing what we were preaching, but we certainly were seeing a lot of patients! That pace of work was ultimately not sustainable for us, but it was helpful. Doing something a lot, figuring out the pace, getting the hang of it, so to speak, is just what that kind of immersion provided. With effort and focus and a lot of enthusiasm, I learned and became comfortable as a doctor. Once we had our first child several years later, we aimed to create a more balanced family life together.

Years later I still welcome all into my practice and do not feel daunted by unusual or extreme pathology nor am I uninterested in common every day ailments, but my enthusiasm has mellowed, my definition of health and help for patients has expanded. I see now that sometimes the patient's illness is difficult to reverse or even entirely irreversible. I see now that not everyone wants to get better. I understand that often what brings a patient to my door is a specific pathology but that in truth, there are other problems more central to their story that need to be addressed. And like most seasoned physicians, I know that some patients I must turn away.

Still, for most, I find ways to help with whatever a patient's complaint might be and even for those who are near to death, I can offer ways to support digestion, improve sleep, decrease itching or shore up the spirits. It is the very variety of patients, the young ones with genetic problems, the teenagers with attitudinal issues, the chronically sick patients in midlife or the older patient hanging on for dear life—for me it is this unpredictable variety of patients scheduled in a day that continues to stretch my knowledge base, stimulate my compassion and inspire me. After decades of practice I find I am calmer, more focused, I get to the central issues of a person's story more efficiently; I derive terrific gratification from the rhythm and straightforwardness of my job and how the years of practice have made it this way.

My receptionist is here when I arrive at the office and a copy of the day's schedule sits on my desk atop my patient charts. A typical day might look like this: (NP= new patient, R= return)

NP : 36 year old woman with allergies and asthma

R : 9 year old boy with ADHD and eczema

R : 47 year old man with high cholesterol and hypertension

NP : 9 month old with sleep issues and repeated ear infections

R : 16 year old boy with cystic acne and attitude problems

R : 22 year old woman with interstitial cystitis and anxiety

R : 39 year old woman with chronic laryngitis and sore throats

NP : 13 year old girl with headaches and painful menstruation

Each new patient is scheduled for an hour and a half, each returning patient for a half hour. I bump one patient up to the next without breaks. Like any good doctor, I wash my hands between patients, as much to stem the spread of germs as to clear my mind and prepare for each patient. I love getting into the rhythm of seeing patients and scheduling long breaks between them interrupts that for me.

I consider it a privilege to be a doctor, to have the opportunity to hear my patients' stories, to understand their illnesses in the context of their lives. There are many things that are essential across the practices of all kinds of medicine, for instance: accurate diagnosis, looking for approaches that will help, doing appropriate referrals and long-term follow-up care. But there are many things that are likely unique about the practice of a naturopathic physician. First of all, though I am interested in whatever the chief complaint is that brought the patient in, I also seek to understand how that issue impacts their life; I want to glean how they individually experience their problems. And as I work overtime to offer help and support to my patients, I want to see that their whole experience of life, from their physical ailments to their mental and emotional health, to their energy level and satisfaction with relationships and work also improve. I would not consider my work a success, for instance, if a patient no longer had laryngitis but was still chronically exhausted. I would not be satisfied if my patient's anxiety improved dramatically but they still suffered tremendously from joint pain and swelling.

As a naturopathic physician I am working to treat the whole person and aiming to do so with the gentlest yet most effective tools at my disposal. I spend a heck of a lot of time encouraging changes to healthier lifestyles including better eating and regular exercise and relaxation. I coach patients and cheer them on as they try new diets to bring down cholesterol, or a new yoga class to ease back pain. I get on the phone and help a new mom get the support she needs to nurse a new baby if the going has been rough. I go online to find smoking cessation programs for patients who are finding quitting the habit insurmountable. I send a letter to a referring physician, explaining my protocol for natural medicine treatment of gastro-esophageal reflux. For some I work as a primary care physician, for others I am a member of their health care team playing my position with commitment and expertise.

On my drive home I am usually listening to the news on the radio or to music, something that allows my mind to wander a bit, and which allow the events and interactions of the day to percolate down through my system. When I finally reach the hustle and bustle of home, my family and evening responsibilities, I am ready.

I get home from work a good hour before my kids and many days quickly change into shorts and tee shirt. I put on my rollerblades, my helmet and grab my son's iPod and head off on the Norwottock Rail Trail. I spend the next 45 minutes rollerblading to my favorite music, dancing in a way, moving my arms, going too fast, getting my heart rate up. After about 3 miles, I come to a slab of granite that has been carved into a bench and inscribed, *Grandpa's Bench,* overlooking a widespread field edged with trees, the Holyoke Range rising sublimely in the distance. I lay there with a sweeping view of the deep blue sky, listening to the cacophony of late afternoon birds, I do my sit-ups, an ab workout my daughter has taught me. Lying on the cold stone, my back dripping with sweat, I am releasing much of the stress of the day. I have come to find solace in the tempo and breeze of skating, in the woods that line this route and the large stretches of water, products of the beaver invasion of the area. The landscape is calming and serene, with dead trees still standing tall, their reflections in the water.

I do try to practice what I preach. I once marveled to a landscape architect friend about how impeccable and inspiring her garden was. She shrugged and said, "Look, I would never go to a doctor who looked really unhealthy, or who seemed like they didn't take care of themselves… it's the same thing, Amy." This was a point well taken. Indeed, I do create time for relaxation and exercise and I do eat well and take a small number of supplements each day. I take time to be with family, and to get away from it all. I owe it to my patients not to hold them to a higher level of discipline and care than I hold myself and I certainly owe that to my family and myself.

We have a tradition around our family table where we share about our days. Sometimes we play *High/Low* where we each talk about a high point and a low point of the day. Sometimes we play *Two Truths & a Lie*, where you recount three things that happened or we experienced that day and everyone else around the table has to guess which event was a lie! Of course, often we just chat. Increasingly, my nearly grown children ask about my patients, about the nature of certain pathologies, about different natural medicine approaches. So much for getting a break from work!

On days when I am not in the clinic, I like many parents, am busy running the household: I spend time buying food, making meals, cleaning, taking care of errands, doing yard work and making phone calls and filling out forms! But I also found early in my work as a doctor that I enjoyed writing about my experiences with patients. I enjoyed sharing my insights about the process of medicine; it was a wonderful counterpoint to seeing patients. Many doctors write, perhaps it is the perfect antidote to the stress of patient care. For me it also allows, even forces me into time for reflection and taking stock. Instead of plowing forward into each new day, I give myself the opportunity to think about what I am doing, what is working, what isn't and how the processes impact me. That I have found an audience of interested readers is a bonus; the process of ruminating and articulating ideas about my experiences and perceptions has intrinsic value to me. Teaching, which I write about in the coming pages is a good companion to writing and

I have found that each has become a fundamental, challenging and essential part of my overall work.

This combination of being a mother and homemaker, seeing patients, writing and teaching, suits me well. I am not doing any one of these things to the point of burnout and each of them naturally and essentially informs and reflects the other parts. I have been tremendously blessed to have a schedule with maximum flexibility, work I love and time to pour affection and attention into both my work and my family.

On Being a Teacher

I seem to have been born to teach. Though I never set out to be an educator, I commonly find myself, in different areas of my life, in positions of leadership or teaching. Often I am surprised by this. I do not think I necessarily know more than others or understand things better. Yet, some confluence of an artist's eye for perception, a modicum of mental clarity, an ability to communicate effectively and probably most essentially, an open personality, often has me educating in the clinical setting, standing before a class of students or before a particular audience or teaching through the written word. I bring a woman and mother's perspective to underline and reinforce ideas and experiences in the world of natural medicine and work to bring back the basic common sense related to healing and wellness.

I was thrown into situations early in my career that required me to be able to stand up in front of a group and share thoughts and knowledge and as the years went by, experience. I was told in naturopathic school that I would *have* to be able to get out there and represent what I did if I wanted people to come to me and that is exactly what I set out to do. In my first years after naturopathic medical school, I lived in Nebraska and did frequent patient education talks where I spoke on everything from preventing winter ailments to first aid care to the treatment of PMS. Young and not especially experienced, I was thrown into settings where individuals wanted to know what I knew. In the late 1980s, there was much less information available about natural medicine approaches. I started lecturing wherever a group would have me—Rotary Clubs, Mother of Twin groups, community colleges, and the local library. People were thirsty for even very basic guidance. This naturally impacted my practice and drew in patients; it also gave me the chance to hone public speaking skills and become comfortable in front of a crowd. I grew to understand that though people want accurate and useful information, they also want to be entertained and inspired.

My husband, Paul and I launched the New England School of Homeopathy in 1990, the first group meeting around our dining room table, with our newborn daughter in tow! Offering long term courses to medical professionals as well as serious lay people, we both have loved. We prefer this format, where we could get to know people, see how different people learn and also inadvertently helping to create community wherever we taught. This had so many advantages over guest lecturing here and there, which I still enjoy doing as well, but it is in the long-term classes where I have found much more satisfaction in the world of teaching. I have consistently taught through NESH in the United States and abroad for the past 20 years, training many individuals and working to create a supportive community along the way. Necessarily then, some of my time is spent in lecture preparation, case write-ups for class work and review of students' work.

In my early years of teaching, as to this day, there is tremendous learning in teaching. When I prepare for a lecture or for any writing, I am better informed on the topic. If I might write about a patient, it sharpens my perceptions as I am taking the history, my ears are perked up so I can explain things more accurately for future readers. I am always thinking to myself, how can I explain this to my students? And in a way, when I am with students in a class room, the questions I am asked help me clarify my thoughts and understanding of what it is I do, day in, day out, with patients.

I recently spoke at a state association for Naturopathic Physician's continuing education. How my profession has grown, hundreds of people were amassed for a weekend's worth of learning, some new to practice while others were seasoned physicians. I knew that my own experience, my own thoughts on the subject matter were valued and that my comfort with my PowerPoint, the cordless mic, the room filled with eager learners helped to put those in attendance at ease, a good place to be when you are trying to learn. By being direct, by speaking with confidence, by citing examples from my own practice and sticking to what I know, I can hopefully inspire others to keep learning, keep seeking ways to help their own patients.

I had the occasion to give the commencement speech at the National College of Naturopathic Medicine (NCNM) in Portland, Oregon, my *alma mater* in the early part of this century. After the ceremony, an older woman came up to me.

She grabbed my arm and pulled me over to a quiet corner. She recounted how she had heard me give a lecture on the Gary Null radio show some 15 years before. As she listened to that show, she became more and more enthralled. By the end of the interview she realized she wanted to do *what I was doing*. She had raised a family and had had a career in an unrelated field. She quit that job and totally changed gears; she began and completed her prerequisite studies, and at long last was accepted at NCNM. And now she had graduated. She came up to thank me for inspiring her so many years before.

I retell this encounter to illustrate how we never know where the seeds we plant will blossom and we never know how experiences we share might impact another person. I have countless emails, postcards and letters from students and colleagues thanking me for some insight or a particular lecture, some are from many years ago. Helping students to see what they do not understand and to be quietly supportive and encouraging and to know them as individuals is work I adore. Watching understanding light up across a person's face is one of the greatest delights a teacher can have; hearing back from someone who feels that their work with me has helped them with their work with a patient is a highlight of any day. I also try to help students figure out what it is that they can best bring to their practice in terms of skills like case taking, listening, being caring. I encourage them to embrace those things they already do well and build upon them while figuring out which things they need more work on.

I have a stack of holiday cards from students that say things like, Thank you for believing in me when I did not believe in myself, thank you for all the time you spent with me when I was struggling with *xyz*, thank you for not being in a rush with me during our clinical work, thank you for guiding me to streamline my caretaking, thank you for modeling balance in your own life, etc. A few years back, Paul and I received a beautiful card from a man we taught in the 1990s. It said simply: "Your work continues to inspire me. My patients have you to thank."

I never set out to be a teacher, but if I have had any positive impact on anyone and that impact has helped lessen another person's suffering, then I have not worked in vain.

On Working with One's Life Partner

I have been in private practice since 1986 with my husband and partner extraordinaire, Paul Herscu. We met on our first day of ND school in the summer of 1982. We did not immediately come together, in fact there were some rocky years between us, but by the end of our education, it was clear we were meant for each other. In Paul I found someone as passionate as I about natural medicine, who also had a terrific sense of humor, an unmatched work ethic, bottomless patience and a kind of deep running grace. His brilliant mind could be put to most any task with creativity and success. He was and remains an original thinker who continues to bring understanding and clarity to the world of homeopathy, systems thinking and how to use our understanding of natural medicine to impact the world of research science and work within the pharmaceutical industry.

To me he brought profound love and acceptance, infusing a level of calmness and direction to my life and our lives together. There was a sureness that in creating a home and life together we would be surrounded by joy, by children, by satisfying work and by the ability to recognize our blessings, although not necessarily in that order! We married on a rain-soaked day in Aloha, Oregon, a handful of hours after our medical school graduation. The skies broke open and cleared to a cerulean blue and the late afternoon sun finally had a moment to shine.

Paul and I are very blessed to have each other in life and in this work. If you met us you would know we have nearly divergent personalities and unique temperaments. I am a people person, I am a morning person, I have very healthy basic habits of living. Paul is a serious and devout student of this and many other arts and a disciplined learner, practitioner and writer. He is encyclopedic in his interests and knowledge of many subject areas and sees connections among and between many of them. I am a book artist and occasionally a cantor, I am committed to physical exercise, healthy eating and getting lots of sleep. We do well with long stretches of time together in quiet or chatting or just working side by side. We have also found ways to be alone and apart especially when work has us on the road. We are both good communicators, remember to do small kindnesses to and for each other and we have fun with each other and among family and friends. On the brink of our empty nest, we will miss the hubbub of a busy family life, but we are looking forward to what the next phase might have in store.

In terms of our patients, when we are stumped with a patient we will see the patient together. If it's my patient, Paul takes the case and if it's his patient, I take the case. This is one of the small gifts we give each other. It is remarkable how a different person asking the same question often gets a totally different response. We can help each other see things more clearly. I have strengths in understanding people and Paul has strengths in understanding remedies though, obviously we are both good at each side of that equation. We love to be at the office together which we do one day a week, we meet in the lunch area for a chat or take a short break together. Paul often sends me his patients that he thinks I will connect with better; I will send him a patient I think he will be more in synch with.

We have always had more work than we can realistically accomplish. Paul can work long hours with little food or sleep. I have often been the one keeping the home fires burning; this division of labor has served us well. On occasion when Paul's time away from me and the family has grown too long, or he is distracted by a compelling realization or understanding, I have had fleeting wishes, like, "Oh, I should have married a person who sells shoes, who would be home at 5 and done!" But alas, I know that being with someone who is engaged and impassioned and ever expanding in his work is imminently interesting and exciting even when simultaneously exhausting. I cannot imagine being with someone who did not at very least *understand* the work I do and in Paul I have a soul mate who truly appreciates all I am and all I do, both in and out of the office.

Chapter 2

Introduction to Pregnancy and Small Children

Motherhood is the Mother of Invention! Babies, Babies, Babies

After two years of marriage, it was time to start thinking about a family. Though we loved our life together in and out of the clinic, my husband and I knew we wanted children and in our late 20s at the time, thought it was as good a time as any to get started. I bought a basal body thermometer and began to wait for day one of my cycle so that we might begin to figure out when I was most fertile. We waited and waited. Waited some more. Turned out I was already pregnant! A bit of a shock, but certainly welcome. I embraced the whole idea of becoming a family, of eating enough protein, of getting regular exercise, of creating a birthing plan to our liking and to thinking about baby names and about how we would handle nursing, diapers, household chores, childcare and work.

There was the birth, a lovely bright-eyed daughter, and two years of getting used to being a mother when the thought seeped through our playroom walls: A sibling, Sophie needs a little brother or sister! So I dug out that thermometer and began to wait for day one of my cycle. We waited and waited. Waited some more. Turned out I was already pregnant. Maybe it was the thermometer!

Now we had a delightful preschooler and a bushy-tailed toddler to chase around. Nursing, diapering, reading picture books, stroller walks, making applesauce, rubbing backs and patting bottoms filled my days. I was adamant about birth control, feeling a bit overwhelmed about the prospect of another child. We thought about a third baby but it was always somewhere down the line, when things calmed down. I was still nursing on demand and had not yet begun to menstruate. So it was with some shock one night, lying in bed, when Misha, at about ten months old, pulled off the breast and scampered over to his papa. I looked down and was frightened by a rather large bump I saw in my lower abdomen. My first thought was, wow, looks like I might just have a fibroid in my uterus. I flipped onto my back. My husband looked down. Our excessively wide opened eyes looked up at each other, we looked down again. A short external exam ensued.

Never even took out the thermometer. When Jonah was born a scant 5 months later (fastest pregnancy on the books!) our growing family was complete.

Perhaps this randomness, this lack of control, this utter not being sure of what happened when, was a metaphor for much there is to know about parenthood. We all like to think we are in control, at least to some extent or another, but in fact, there is much that is out of our hands even when best laid plans are made and especially with regard to childrearing.

We embraced these children, built a life around them, created community where we lived and leaned on it when needed. My husband's first book, *The Homeopathic Treatment of Children, Pediatric Constitutional Types* published in 1991, had received wide acclaim and our practice was filling up with all sorts of children—those who were robust but perhaps had an issue with allergies or eczema to those brought in with more severe neurological, psychological, physiological or chromosomal issues. Our own brood at home kept us busy; there truly was never a dull moment. A love affair with children, our children, children in our lives and children in our practice had begun.

Whenever I attend a baptism or baby naming or baby welcoming ceremony I am struck with the hopefulness that daring to bring a child into this world reflects. I am sure I felt that to a degree before I had kids, but now that my three children are raised, I feel it with a quiet, but well-earned certainty. The job description at least in this culture, at this time—birth this helpless baby, raise her with unending love and care, spend sleepless nights, angst ridden hours, endure deep uncertainty or bottomless pride, and then, then launch them from the nest, gently prod them out of the house, cut them loose–is bizarre. Into what else in our lives to we pour our hearts and souls, hours and hours not to mention endless resources and then push away? Yet that is even, I dare say, how we know we have done our job well. We hope for the confident, kind, capable person emerging on the other end of 18 or 20 or 25 years, off into the world to offer and embrace what they may.

The wisdom, advice, strategies or techniques I share with patients on everything from nighttime sleeping and diapering to weaning or discipline comes from experience, both with my own and with hundreds of families in my practice. One of the things I love best is to work with a family on health issues and also to support parents in helping create the most harmonious households they can, to create space for siblings to get along, to parent effectively the particular child with their particular idiosyncrasies, their talents, their personality, their individual temperament. Nothing works for everyone although good and open communication, clarity and consistency do go a far way with most every family I know.

I do not know what I would have done without a medical training and a natural medicine background while raising my family. In terms of prevention, in terms of treatment, in terms of staying calm in the face of emergency, I am ever thankful that I was able to bring into the raising of my family knowledge from my professional world. In the pages that follow you will read about babies and children and teenagers and some of the unique ways they present for this practitioner of natural medicine. Hopefully you can pick up some tips and enjoy the stories!

Infertility

When Rachael came to see me, referred by a student of mine, it was the middle of a busy day. I had seen several return patients and a few with acute problems and one other new patient. It was after lunch and I felt renewed and mentally clear. Her problem was in some ways very simple, in other ways a challenge. She desperately wanted to get pregnant. At 38 she felt her doorway to birthing a child was narrowing and her fertility specialist agreed. She has already spent four years trying hormonal treatments, intrauterine insemination, and *in vitro* fertilization. She and her husband were at their wits' end and came to me as a last resort.

Many in the world of natural medicine see fertility as another general reflection of overall health. Most women in good health eventually conceive, but for some reason or reasons, some do not. There was nothing perceptibly wrong with Rachael and of course her husband had been examined and had a sperm count and morphology that was within normal limits.

I am always clear with these patients that I cannot treat them for their infertility. I can try to do those things that will optimize the environment for them to conceive. I often encourage my patients to continue with their fertility treatments if their doctors are willing. It can happen that previously attempted strategies work after naturopathic and/or homeopathic care.

With Rachael, I felt that she was basically in good health. I did a complete review of systems with her and we spoke about the big stressors in her life. She was happily married and worked as a third grade teacher. She was an avid exerciser and helped to take care of aging parents. She put a lot of pressure on herself to do a good job, to look good and to keep a nice home.

She was overinvested it seemed to me with her weight, her diet and her appearance. She obsessed about the extra five pounds she thought she was carrying and about how her hair never looked right. She tended to become irritable, especially with her husband when she was feeling down on herself. In the physical realm, she struggled with constipation and ensuing hemorrhoids. She had certain characteristics that brought to mind the homeopathic remedy *Sepia officinalis*, which of all things, is made from the ink of the cuttlefish. This remedy, long used by homeopaths, has helped patients, especially women, when there is a kind of stagnation of the blood or a kind of lethargy in any of the systems. It also so happens that inability to get pregnant is also something that this remedy has helped, both for those women who are unable to get pregnant and those who historically have been unable to carry a baby to term. This is certainly not the only remedy to use in these situations and it is not a linear sort of prescription, that is, infertility equals needing the remedy *Sepia*. It will only be prescribed when the rest of the person also fits the remedy, therein lies the greatest challenge to the homeopath!

I prescribed *Sepia officinalis* to Rachel and lo and behold she conceived that very first month. I will never know if the remedy is what enabled her to get pregnant and give birth to a wonderful, big and healthy baby girl, but I can guarantee you this: Rachael thinks that's what did it. She has sung my praises to many infertile friends, some of whom have made it to my doors wanting the same treatment. But not every woman who does not conceive will necessarily get pregnant with a natural medicine approach. There is much we do not yet understand about conception and carrying babies to term.

In fact, one of my least favorite complaints to treat in my practice is infertility. For many couples having difficulty, carrying a child would be the only outcome that would be perceived as positive. Meanwhile, I have worked with women who never did conceive, but have become headache free, or are now sleeping better, no longer have irritable bowel syndrome or have lost a lifelong tendency for depression. Hopefully in situations like this, there is also openness to adoption, as there are so many children in need and so many arms made for loving. I aim to be very clear with my patients in this category, that it is my sincere hope that they do get pregnant, but also, I want to see that they feel better in general, that other physical body symptoms recede and that their moods and spirits are moved in a positive direction.

Rachel was not satisfied with one child and yearned for a sibling for her toddler. When she came to me seeking another "dose of that stuff," I was a bit reluctant. I told her it's not always so easy, we would need to do the same thing, take her full story and prescribe from there. Rachael decided that if she did get pregnant and if she did carry the baby to term and if the baby was a girl, her name would be Amy. Sure enough little Amy was born three years after her sister; this duo keep their contented mother busy and have brought endless joy along with all the overwhelm small children spawn in their wake, into her life. But for every story I have like this, I have others of women who never conceive. So, should women try natural medicine and homeopathy in particular for help and support? Sure. Is it always effective? No.

Pregnancy

Ah, to be pregnant, full of life, aglow with the lofty purpose of carrying a child into this world! But what if this image of beauty and saintliness crashes and becomes one of constipation, exhaustion, sore breasts, heartburn, backache and varicose veins? What if the smell of your husband's breath sends you running to the bathroom, or if your face gets so full you feel unrecognizable. And that shiny hair and gorgeous skin, what if instead you have a dark rash across your cheeks and your hair seems unnecessarily greasy? All your dreams of the wonderful glowing pregnancy might be met with another chapter. Natural medicine is made to order! Working gently on mom and without harm to baby, I prescribe gentle remedies and approaches for a pregnant woman's acute problems as well as their overall constitutional health.

I spend a fair amount of time in any visit I have with a pregnant woman emphasizing the following basic areas:

1. Proper nutrition. I focus especially on adequate intake of foods rich in calcium and protein. I tell moms-to-be to enjoy what they love but to also remember daily doses of fruits and vegetables and plenty of water. I encourage the patient to take prenatal vitamins. Some of the known problems that arise due to malnutrition, such as neural tube defects related to folic acid deficiency, occur before most women even know they are pregnant. Nonetheless, it is wise to help the patient find a prenatal vitamin that agrees with her digestively speaking, and to remind her to stick with it throughout the pregnancy as well as during lactation.

2. Proper rest. I talk about how growing a baby is a full-time job on top of whatever else the woman may be juggling; all that work, with no extra rest, will lead to sure exhaustion. The extra rest must be worked in, either by going to bed earlier, rising later and/or napping.

3. The importance of exercise. This would not be a time to give up the exercise plan. For those having a vaginal birth, it will help enormously if the muscles of the body are in good shape and the lungs as well, because giving birth

is an aerobic and physical marathon of sorts. For those with scheduled Cesarean section, this advice still holds, as women in better shape will have more resources to marshal during convalescence from that major surgery. A half-hour stroll is enough. Classes designed specifically for the pregnant woman, such as prenatal yoga, stretching, or water aerobics can also be fun while helping some women begin to connect with other mothers-to-be. I will get on the phone while a patient is with me or on the Internet and help locate something they can afford that is nearby that sounds appealing. I encourage them to find something early on, before they get so big that they might feel self-conscious or uncomfortable.

4. Feeling good about the birthing plan and care team. I try to touch on the importance of this with all my pregnant patients. The surest way to put a labor into stop mode is if, at the time of the birth, the mother is not comfortable with the environment or people in it. I encourage my mothers and their partners to consider their options carefully and to make changes when necessary up to and including at the actual time of the birth.

5. Finding support at home and work. It is essential to get enough and the right type of support during the pregnancy itself as well as after the baby arrives. This might be through paid helpers or with family and friends filling in. Troubleshooting with a partner or friend as to where my new mom may most need support and then getting it in place can help head off many physical and psychological problems before they have a chance to arise.

Many women come to me seeking constitutional homeopathic care before or during a pregnancy. Sometimes I agree that it is a good idea. Here are some general guidelines I think about when deciding whether to give a pregnant patient a constitutional homeopathic remedy.

If the patient had difficult past pregnancies with regard to physical issues like morning sickness, digestive upset, constipation, skin problems, vaginal infections, musculo-skeletal complaints, etc., I always recommend the patient seek constitutional homeopathic care *before* conception if possible or at least during the first trimester. In this way, I hope to help her head off any unnecessary problems with the pregnancy so that she may enjoy this special time of life, without all the nuisances that get in the way.

If the patient has had other children with chronic problems like allergies, eczema, ongoing infections, asthma, digestive complaints, attention deficit hyperactivity disorder, or autistic spectrum disorders, I recommend that both parents seek constitutional treatment before conception. If that's not feasible, I recommend constitutional treatment during pregnancy for the mother. Many health problems *do* run in families; for instance, having one autistic child greatly increases your chances of having another. Certainly we see allergies running in families as well. By treating the parent(s) constitutionally, I hope to reduce the chances that a subsequent child will be likewise affected.

If the chief complaint is morning sickness, I only offer treatment if it is severe, if it is long lasting (through the day or beyond the first trimester), or if the patient has a history of severe, protracted morning sickness in a previous pregnancy. I do not treat low-grade nausea as it reflects a certain health of the pregnancy—those hormones of early pregnancy circulating and wreaking havoc are normal. Instead, I encourage the mother to use other approaches, most importantly, to eat whatever she likes, whenever she likes it. Salty crackers help many.

In fact, it is often quite easy to find a homeopathic remedy for a pregnant woman because for most, the life-energy is in a heightened state, and symptoms and cravings are often clear and specific. Strong food desires, new sleep positions, extreme body temperatures, and personality quirks appear for many women during pregnancy, giving especially the homeopath much fodder to help choose an appropriate homeopathic remedy.

In addition to whenever else I may have seen a woman during the pregnancy, I like to see my pregnant gals about a month before they are due. At this visit, I address any concerns they may have about their current health as well as questions about the upcoming labor and delivery. If they are experiencing no particular health problems, I may give a dose of the constitutional remedy as a way of strengthening the patient in preparation for childbirth. Provided there are no extenuating circumstances or illnesses in the child, I love to see the baby in the first month sometime, to get a sense of the baby constitutionally, to check in with mom, especially for the first time mothers, and to see how the nursing or feeding relationship is coming along.

Ugliest Legs This Side of the Mississippi: A Case of Painful Varicose Veins in Pregnancy

A long-term patient of mine had always responded well to the constitutional remedy *Lycopodium* for premenstrual syndrome and a lifelong tendency toward constipation. Over the course of her first pregnancy and with the impact of a waitressing job where she spent six to eight hours a day on her feet, her varicose veins had worsened. Now in the sixth month of her second pregnancy, the veins were intolerable. She reported pain and swelling in her legs and a kind of deep aching. She mentioned in passing that, "Yup, I now have the ugliest legs this side of the Mississippi!"

In homeopathy, as in other professions, we have certain tools of the trade. In this business we use a book, which has now been put into computer program format, called a repertory. A repertory lists all the symptoms known to humanity and the homeopathic remedies that have been known to help with those particular symptoms. We are able to utilize this resource to help us coordinate and streamline our understanding of a patient's symptoms, hopefully without getting overwhelmed.

For the patient at hand, if we look in the repertory under the symptoms, 'Extremities, Varices, Pregnancy, during,' we find *Lycopodium* as one of the remedies listed, that is, this symptom has been helped by this remedy in others. Because I had known this remedy to help her so dramatically in the past, I prescribed it again. I was pretty confident about the prescription because she seemed much like she had always seemed: a bit insecure, somewhat anxious about her family, the pregnancy and her work. She also continued to crave sweets, had deep fatigue in the late afternoon, and often felt bloated—all common and descriptive symptoms of people who have done well with the remedy *Lycopodium*.

So, I was surprised when she returned to my office two weeks later reporting no improvement—in fact, she was worse.

I needed to take a more complete case, which then revealed that the veins were incredibly painful and quite sensitive to touch. This sensitivity was so great that the support hose she dutifully wore were almost unbearable. She also said that pain in the veins was rather stinging. She had simultaneously developed varicosities around the vulvar area as well with large bluish veins that were also stinging and painful. I went back to consulting my repertory again and found the following helpful symptoms or rubrics:

Extremities, Varices, leg, painful

Extremities, Varices, leg, pregnancy

Extremities, Varices, leg, sensitive

Female Genitalia, Veins, varicose

This combination of specific symptoms having to do with the veins, especially during pregnancy, with such a specific sensation as stinging, pointed strongly to the remedy *Hamamelis virginiana* (Witch hazel), which I prescribed. This remedy is not as commonly prescribed as *Lycopodium* and I was less familiar with it. When used in the world of botanical medicine, we see *Hamamelis* utilized for issues of constipation, varicosities and liver complaints. Some homeopathic remedies were initially utilized based on their botanical medicine indications, and this is one like that.

She called the next week to report that though her legs still looked pretty bad, the pain was much reduced and she could work without the terrible aching. I suggested she wait and take no more *Hamamelis* at that time. During the eighth month of pregnancy, I gave her *Hamamelis* again, when the stinging and discomfort had picked up. Stopping work about three weeks before her due date and getting into the local pool an hour a day to walk in the water, helped. I suggested that as a way to massage the legs and push the fluids back into the vessels. I also reminded her to salt her food to taste, which helps to keep the blood in the vessels, but only during pregnancy! The delivery and postnatal period were uneventful, and though this patient likes to brag about her ugly legs, they no longer cause her any discomfort.

So send your pregnant friends and relatives to homeopaths for gentle, effective, and safe treatment of common problems of pregnancy—and to treat or prevent worse problems, based on family history. This is one time of life when most any woman can benefit from this kind of care.

Tips for New Moms and Families

I remember fondly the years of tending to little ones. Having three kids in three and a half years would not be my recommendation to most sane people, but it did afford me the opportunity of 'total surrender!' We had our good days and bad, weeks of cabin fever in the dead of New England winter, whole months it seems given over to chicken pox or runny noses; lots of time making discoveries in our backyard, figuring out how machines work, how to communicate effectively and with kindness, exploring the wonders of reading, doing art projects, baking, cooking, cleaning and playing with friends. Each child is a gift through which *we* keep on opening, through love and acceptance, laughter and understanding and ultimately, letting go. Natural medicine and homeopathy allow us to address the bumps and bruises along the way—from the throes of colic, to the adolescent PMS—I am ever thankful to have these tools both at the office to help the young families in my practice, as well as in my home.

Here are some general recommendations I make, especially for nursing mothers:

Tending to baby and mom: The first 8-10 days after the baby is home, the mom should be in bed most of the day tending to the baby, with her partner, friend, doula, support person or perhaps her own mother tending to her. Let others do the housework, care for siblings, do the laundry, shop and cook. This reduces the chance of the mother getting a post-partum infection or mastitis, and allows her to recover from the experience of childbirth and to bond with the baby.

Getting help: If resources are available, I ask the parents to figure out what is most needed and then hire good people. If the mom likes being with the baby, have the helper do the things she doesn't care to do. If what she needs is an hour at the gym, or if she prefers to grocery shop and do some domestic chores herself, then let the helper take the baby out for a walk in the stroller or in a baby carrier. If mom has to get right back to work, figure out how to optimize time for bonding with baby.

If money is scarce: I have the parents look to friends or family to give the help most needed—doing laundry, preparing meals. For the latter I remind families to ask for food in volume and things that can be frozen for later use and without being rude, asking for things you actually like! It might make most sense to have helpers give focused attention to older siblings. I really emphasize the following maxim: Forget the idea of trying to do it all yourself! The whole idea of mom and/or dad or partner home alone raising the kids and keeping the household running was never a very good one. It leads to burnout, to feeling overwhelmed, anxious, and inadequate. I tell new parents, "Show me a mom who hasn't thought once or twice about getting in the car and just driving away, and I'll show you a mom who doesn't know how to drive!"

Caring for yourself: Drink plenty of water and try to eat well. Many new mothers find it difficult to take care of themselves while taking care of the baby, but I remind them that they will be more loving and effective parents if well fed, rested and exercised!

Getting out of the house: After the first few weeks, it is important to try getting out of the home every day—with or without the baby—even if just to do errands or meet a friend for tea. This will help the parents to preserve their mental health. I encourage all new parents in my practice to make and keep a date with their partner—bring the baby along if you must, but get out of the house for some adult time away from the endless work of keeping house and tending to little ones! It gives parents a chance to reconnect with each other.

Finding supportive role models: Seek the advice of, and spend time with other moms and parents you admire. Avoid people in your life who are critical of you or not supportive. This is your baby to raise as you see appropriate.

Letting the emotions run: Sudden weeping or uncontrollable laughter is not uncommon; these emotional swings are part and parcel of the hormonal ride of having a new baby. Note that this is true for new parents of adopted children as well. That said, true postpartum depression must be addressed under the care of a qualified health care provider, for the safety of mother and baby alike.

Nursing/pumping milk: For those mothers going right back to work, I encourage nursing or pumping milk for at least 3-6 months, if at all possible. This will be very healthy for your baby and for the mother/baby relationship. I stress this even more if older children in the family have had allergies or asthma. If it's not possible, don't worry—many of us were never nursed and we seem to be thriving! Hopefully, your work situation will allow you to be home when you need to be, and those you work for and with will be supportive of your new role as parent.

Lowering expectations: I always encourage my new moms to aim low, setting very small goals for each day that will be possible to reach. Children grow up fast, and savoring even the mundane is itself a goal.

Choosing Homeopathy for Children

There are so many choices to make as parents these days. Natural childbirth or not? To nurse or bottle feed? Cloth diapers or disposable? Family bed or crib? How many years between children? What type of preschool or schooling? The choices and options for many families in our times are endless. So, too, for the kind of medical care to use. How much is safe to treat at home? When is it imperative to get the opinion of a trained medical professional? What if my partner and I don't agree?

In my decades of practice I have had the pleasure of working with many families, offering natural medicine choices for health care issues. Some patients come to me already certain they want to go the natural way. Others come in not really knowing the type of work I do as a naturopathic physician specializing in homeopathy. But they know someone who was helped with a similar problem, so they want the same assistance. Still others arrive quite skeptical, having been disappointed by previous therapies and attempts to help their child and almost desperate for help.

I have always been pleased to be able to offer a non-toxic, effective and gentle approach to first-aid, acute and chronic health issues that arise in the course of raising a family. For most first-aid and acute conditions, in the vast majority of situations, there are wonderful at-home treatments available such as hydrotherapy, massage and approaches related to nutrition and herbal medicines. In addition, a limited number of homeopathic remedies are used over and over again including: *Aconite, Belladonna, Pulsatilla, Chamomilla, Sulphur, Arnica, Mercurius* and *Arsenicum album*. I truly do not know where I would be as a physician without these medicines and as a mother without these dear friends on the medicine cabinet shelf.

Thankfully, there are wonderful books on acute homeopathic prescribing written in a way that enables a parent to choose the correct remedy for things like bee stings, sore throats, teething and diarrhea. Most of these books will also caution parents as to when it is essential to seek further medical care. No one wants to put a child at risk because of a philosophical belief in natural treatment. There is a time and a place for all types of medicine.

For children with chronic illness, constitutional homeopathy offers one type of approach that addresses the underlying causes of the illness and hopefully presents solutions to difficult physical, emotional, behavioral and psychological problems. In constitutional treatment (for both children and adults), we give a homeopathic remedy for the whole person—their physical, mental and emotional state.

I spend a fair amount of time trying to help people understand what it is I do and how I work. I take as much time as is necessary for the parent to learn that all aspects of the child will be important to me. I need to understand not just the particular diagnosis, but also how they experience their problem in all the minute details. I need to understand little things, like what and how they eat and how they sleep; things related to temperament and personality, like how they behave with new children or if they're more of a leader or a follower. I explain how I will be interested in the mother's pregnancy and in the child's earliest months, their development as well as their experience of school and their social lives.

We try to put the child's illnesses into the context of the rest of their lives and understand them in a complete way. Naturally, I will be observing the relationship between parent and child, how clingy they are, how they respond to limit-setting, how they communicate with each other—all of these are important to prescribing the correct remedy to help the child with whatever complaint caused the parent to make the appointment.

For this sort of constitutional homeopathic care, it is good to have an objective person prescribe (i.e., not the parent!) and to follow the child over time. During constitutional care, some homeopaths will ask that the child not be treated at home for first-aid or acute conditions so as not to interfere with their treatment—other practitioners may feel fine about home care.

So whether your child is prone to first-aid or acute illnesses or has a more chronic disease, having homeopathy more available than ever before, gives many families the choice of using this safe and effective approach.

Wrap Up Those Babies!

Sarah, a young mother, called me one morning during autumn. Her adorable 18 month-old daughter, Leslie, seemed to be getting sick. Sarah was concerned because she was pregnant again, and feeling very tired and under the weather herself. She hoped that whatever Leslie was brewing would not also affect her.

I had treated Leslie over the course of her first year for colic and sleep problems, using the homeopathic remedy *Calcarea carbonica*. A robust and hearty child, she was full of smiles, curious and strong-willed. She had her mother's beautiful red hair and light green eyes with a pale complexion. I asked Sarah what was going on now. She said her daughter had a low-grade fever and that her face was flushed; she was crying off and on and generally in a bad mood. Leslie had not had a bowel movement that day or the day before, which was uncommon for her. She seemed mad and irritable and was difficult to please.

I asked Sarah what had been going on the last few days. Had they been around other sick children? Were there any extenuating circumstances that Sarah thought I should know about? Understanding the context is certainly important for making a good prescription in more challenging chronic complaints, but it can also be very useful for acute prescriptions as well.

Sarah recalled that her husband had taken Leslie on a long bike ride the day before. Leslie was secured in the baby seat and wearing her helmet, but Sarah had been worried because the day had grown chilly and breezy, and they had been out for several hours.

This is not an uncommon story —ailments from exposure to the cold or from exposure to wind. It may not have been an unusually windy day, but the wind generated by the moving bicycle could create a certain stress on a passenger riding in the back, especially if the individual is susceptible. A *Calcarea carbonica* child like Leslie might easily slip into an acute illness if certain stressors were strong enough.

There are many homeopathic remedies to consider when a patient falls ill from an exposure to wind, such as *Aconite, Belladonna, Bryonia, Hepar sulphuricum,* and *Silicea.* Still other remedies are indicated when a patient gets ill after exposure to cold. This tough little girl, in typical *Calcarea carbonica* constitutional style, had worked up quite a sweat, especially on her head, during the first part of the ride in the warmer part of the day. But then the temperatures dropped and the sun hid behind clouds. The wind blowing on her damp head for over an hour, coupled with the general coldness of the afternoon, simply stressed Leslie's little system too much.

This day of our phone call, I could hear Leslie howling in the background. I gathered more information about her current presentation: She had a dryness to her, even though she was feverish. Her head was hot and her extremities were cold, and she was flushed, with large wide-open pupils.

Each of these observances pointed to the homeopathic remedy *Belladonna,* which is a wonderful tool we have for treating all sorts of inflammatory processes, especially in the early stages where perhaps the inflammation has not yet settled onto one organ or organ system. Homeopaths also know from experience that when constitutional *Calcarea carbonica* patients develop an acute illness, *Belladonna* is often indicated.

I asked Sarah to give Leslie one dose of *Belladonna* 30c and to call me or bring her daughter into the office that afternoon if she was not better. It was reasonable to think that Leslie had either an earache or some other beginning inflammatory process going on somewhere—hence the fever alongside the irritability.

Sarah called back a few hours later to say that Leslie had fallen asleep moments after taking the remedy and had woken up back to her perky self. I did see them in the office two days later to check Leslie's ears and listen to her lungs, which were clear.

I encourage the parents in my practice to take their little ones on all sorts of outings: bike rides, walks in the stroller, hikes in the backpack, but especially for those kids that would be more susceptible, I also remind parents to cover the ears and be sure the weather is not going to be too much of a stress.

Colic: The Curse of the Newborn

There is nothing more miraculous than bringing a baby into the world. To have the opportunity to raise a child and create a family is one of the greatest blessings there is in life. Children come to us one after another in rapid succession, or perhaps after years of planning, or as surprises later-in-life, by giving birth to them or through the hard work and miracle of adoption. Regardless, sometimes things go smoothly those first few months and sometimes things are a little rockier.

When a baby has colic, and is uncomfortable or in pain, especially for first time parents, the whole experience can be overwhelming and can make parents feel powerless, insecure and frustrated. Parents wish that baby came with directions, which unfortunately, he or she does not! Natural medicine can help with colic and in turn can help families get back to the lofty and sometimes mundane business of loving and caring for baby, which even with the most easy-going child, can be exhausting. In this chapter, I will share a bit about the homeopathic and naturopathic treatments for colic.

Colic is defined in the Merck Manual as "a symptom complex of early infancy characterized by paroxysms of crying apparently due to abdominal pain and irritability." I have also seen colic described in medical texts as "paroxysmal fussing of infancy," which perhaps better describes the problem. Colic begins some time in the first few weeks and for most babies, it does not last beyond the fourth month or so. Most infants with colic continue to gain weight well, and may seem extremely hungry. The constant or intermittent crying can lead the baby to swallow much air, which exacerbates matters with regard to gas and abdominal bloating.

By the time a family appears at my office for the treatment of colic, they are generally in a desperate state, worn out, sleep-deprived, overwhelmed by feelings of inadequacy and at the end of the rope. I do remind parents that colic will not last, but that hopefully we can find an approach which will help bring baby back to balance quickly, so that the child can focus on the work of eating, sleeping, learning and growing in a more peaceful and calm way.

As far as other natural medicines go, I recommend some of the following:

If mom is nursing, I ask her to try to drink some non-alcoholic beer a half hour or so before nursing; perhaps due to the hops in it, it may help *her* to relax. This can help to break the cycle of a crying baby which leads mother to being very nervous, which doesn't help baby.

I will also show mom and partner some basic baby massage that works to help baby relax. I may recommend a baby massage class if there is a local one handy. It is also terrific for encouraging bonding with the baby.

I may model, especially for first time parents whose own parents may not be around various ways of holding, rocking and swaddling baby. Sometimes a little one just likes it a certain way and it takes time to figure that out. Some infants respond well to music or to background noise. As with other conditions I may recommend the family visit a cranial osteopath for treatment which often helps colic.

Chamomile, mint and fennel tea are all carminative, meaning that they reduce the formation of gas. It is safe to give baby one to two ounces of tea per day. Make it with hot water as you would for a cup of tea and let it cool. In a baby that is strictly nursing, it can be difficult to get this into a child, but for those who also take a bottle, this is fine to try.

And I will always encourage parents who are bottle feeding, to simply try a different formula. There are idiosyncratic ways babies respond to milk; it may not be a true allergy, but they may do better with cow dairy or with soy or with goat milk. Try swaddling your baby—it provides a nice snug feeling; some may like it, for others it will be torture!

I also work with some parents on approaches to overall stress reduction, if it seems possible. For some, it seems like adding one more thing would just be more stressful!

Sometimes the baby will do better if the nursing mother avoids *Brassicaceae* (broccoli, cauliflower, kale, etc), and dairy, as well as onions and garlic. If the mother comes to me having already tried this to no effect, I tell her to resume her normal diet and I go to work looking for the best homeopathic remedy for the baby.

It is important to remember that any homeopathic remedy can be indicated for a baby suffering from colic. I always take a complete case no matter what the complaint. I try to understand everything there is to know about the colic-when it's worse, what seems to make the baby feel better or worse and what the baby's bowel habits are. I also like to know other general information about the mother's pregnancy and the little one's birth and delivery. I will ask about the baby's skin, urination, room temperature preferences, and sleep position and habits. I then try to see how these physical elements fall into the child's overall temperament and mood. I prescribe for the whole child with a special eye to the digestive discomfort.

The main homeopathic remedies I use for the treatment of colic and their indications follow:

Chamomilla is used when the baby cries often and cannot be comforted. They are restless, seem angry and may arch their back in effort to find a comfortable position. This remedy has done much to introduce parents to homeopathy and to offer help when needed. The stools are often green and offensive smelling, even in the breastfed baby.

The *Pulsatilla* baby develops hiccoughs soon after eating and you can hear rumbling from the belly. This is the infant that though not comfortable, *is* consolable and feels best when in mother's arms being held or gently rocked. In Caucasian babies, you will commonly be able to see a fine marbled look to the skin, with visible small veins on the face. *Pulsatilla* little ones in general, are thirstless, so do not be thrown off by the baby that wants to nurse or have the bottle for hours on end, it is the comfort associated with feeding that they crave more than the actual fluid.

The baby that needs *Nux vomica* will most often also be constipated. They will need to push very hard for each bowel movement, even if the stool is soft or mushy. They will really want to be kept warm and will be angry about most of what one does in trying to help them. They may also have a stuffy nose and get frustrated with that as well.

Lycopodium babies have a look of anxiety about them, with a wrinkled brow and worried expression. They suffer from trapped gas and seem to worsen in the late afternoon or early evening just as everyone in the family seems to be getting most irritable. They can be helped with a warm compress or warm hot water bottle held to the belly and will always feel better if they can pass gas. They may also have cracks behind the ears, a bit of eczema cropping up here and there.

I will prescribe *Colocynthis* when the main modality is that the baby is better with firm pressure to the abdomen; when the parents report that they must hoist the baby up and over their shoulder and allow that sort of pressure to relieve the pain and crying.

A *Magnesium phosphoricum* baby's colic is helped if they can keep their knees up by the chest, which seems to relieve the bloating and gas; they will also settle down some if they can have a good burp.

I do think about the remedy *Ignatia* for a baby with troubling colic, especially if the mother had experienced a grief, such as a loss of another baby in the past or loss of her own mother or husband during pregnancy. These emotional events in the mother's life influence the baby at hand.

I most often give the remedy in a 30c potency, one time, and ask the parent to report back to me in a week. I will make follow-up prescriptions based on how the baby has done.

Using some of these gentle natural medicine approaches has allowed me to help many a family in need and bring those sweet smiles and little cooing sounds back into the nursery. When mom feels less stressed by a crying and inconsolable baby, it's amazing how much more she can get done and how much happier everyone in the household is!

Once I have come to a prescription for the colic I ask if there are any other things the mother or other parent are concerned with and try to give advice accordingly.

Chapter 3

For the Children in Your Life

Are You Giving Too Many Medicines to People in Your Family? Remember: Less is More!

Some years ago, my younger sister had her first child. This new beautiful addition to our family was such a wonderful and welcome event and one that, as the doctor in the family, allows me to play a special role. From other new moms in my practice I get to hear and respond to all those worries and questions at all hours of the day and night! I hear questions about babies like, what to do about incessant crying, difficulty with sleep, bothersome rashes, runny noses, challenges with nursing, etc. I also have had questions from new mothers about shifts in digestion, problems with breastfeeding and issues around moodiness and irrational worry. While I'm on the phone, the grandmother or uncle from the 'other side' might throw in a question or two about their recent health concerns, while they have me on the line!

I debate long and hard when a baby is born to a family member, someone in my circle of friends or to a patient's family whether to recommend or gift that family a homeopathic first aid kit. At first glance, it seems that every family should have one, that it will make giving a remedy at home that much easier. Or, if I am prescribing by telephone for an acute situation, the remedies will be right at hand. But that quick and easy access to remedies might not always be the best thing. There is something tempting about 'fixing' all the little problems or to trying to 'nip things in the bud.' With new mothers and fathers who might not have the experience of weathering the common ups and downs of the first few years in life, I have found that education and encouragement are oftentimes more indicated than homeopathic remedies. This debate has had me come up with the following general thoughts on this topic:

When it's *not* a good idea to treat acute situations at home with homeopathic remedies:

1. When they are severe or life threatening, the best place for the child is with those who are expert at treating emergencies, that is, in the hospital. We cannot be wed to our medical/philosophical beliefs when a child's life is in danger. We can always go back to natural medicine once the child is safe. It is fine to use a remedy on the way, or while under allopathic care.
2. While your child is under constitutional care. If any acute prescribing is going to be done during constitutional care, it should be done in consultation with the prescribing practitioner. The reason for this is that oftentimes the acute situation can offer insight and information to the homeopath as to the ongoing treatment of the child. If the parents or others run to give remedies with each set of symptoms, it can:
    a. Actually confuse the case for the practitioner and,

b. Deny the practitioner potentially useful information about the way that child either reacted to the remedy or manifests acute illness, both important bits of data that go into case analysis and long term follow-up care.

This is especially true for the child who is being treated for mental or emotional conditions like anxiety, depression or OCD, ADHD, or autism spectrum disorders, seizure disorders or any other kind of chronic illness. In these cases, having symptoms shift around or toward the physical plane while the rest of the child improves may lead a homeopath to counsel the family that enduring those symptoms or offering non-homeopathic palliative or allopathic care may be the indicated route.

3. If you find you are giving remedies - either the same one or different ones – frequently, every week or several times per month, it would mean to me that this child had certain patterns of illness and susceptibility and would instead benefit from constitutional care.

4. If the problem is something that would pass on its own, is not long-lasting or severe I would not give a remedy. Of course it is difficult to know early on in an illness if it is going to be long lasting or not. It will not hurt the child to have a cold, a minor cough, a passing skin rash or to be cranky for few days. My goal is that all of the children I treat develop healthy immune systems, something that occasional, not-too-serious viral illnesses helps them to do. I also want parents in my care to learn how to meet the emotional and physical needs of their children by trying many approaches, not only giving homeopathic remedies.

5. I would not recommend giving remedies to siblings of sick children 'just so they can have some, too.' There are some who do prescribe prophylactically during an epidemic of some sort, but that is a matter for another time.

The underlying thought here is that the remedies do act and can have an impact. Most of us would not routinely offer our children or prescribe for our patients pharmaceutical products to be taken frequently or at the presence of any fleeting symptom. Homeopathic remedies need to be treated with the same sort of care and respect.

When it's a good idea to treat acute situations:

1. When you've tried other natural, gentle approaches and they have not worked.
2. When you know that a particular set of prodromal symptoms for the child in question always lead to the same problem and you can catch it early.
3. When you are working with a qualified practitioner and they recommend it.
4. When your child is not being treated constitutionally and the acute problems are infrequent.
5. When all of the above is true, it is good to offer a remedy when the symptoms themselves are clear and you can prescribe with at least a degree of confidence.

After reading this, I imagine that many of you will feel guilty, that perhaps you have over-prescribed for those you love. Not to worry, it rarely will lead to any severe problems, emotional issues or any sort of toxic, overdose symptoms. The worst that happens is that the overall case is muddied for the homeopath. What we are looking for in our recommendations to family and friends is a balanced posture towards the prescribing of homeopathic remedies. Use them carefully when they are indicated and use them well. But many may want to put that homeopathic first aid kit a little higher on the bathroom shelf so that you will be less often tempted to grab a remedy at the first sign of any sickness. As to my sister, I will probably wind up giving her that first aid kit after all, to have on hand, to dust off once in a while, when a remedy is truly indicated.

Homeopathy and Natural Medicine Help One Girl Step Up to the Plate!

An adorable and bright 13 year old girl, Laila, was brought to see me for the treatment of severe gastritis. About a year before our first visit, she had an injury to her shoulder, though neither she nor the parents remembered what had happened to it. She came home from school complaining of pain and several days later she was taken to the pediatrician who recommended keeping an eye on it. After almost a month of pain and discomfort, as well as x-ray diagnostic work, visits to a chiropractor as well as an osteopathic physician, no gross physical abnormalities were detected. Adjustments, massage and other forms of bodywork were tried to no avail. In due time, Laila was prescribed a regimen of non-steroidal, anti-inflammatory medications, which she took faithfully and which took the edge off of the pain, but did not totally relieve it; Laila began to complain of stomachaches.

After several months on these medications for her shoulder and with increasing discomfort in the digestive tract, she was diagnosed with gastro-esophageal reflux. Her family physician recommended she discontinue the anti-inflammatory medicines. She was then prescribed drugs for the acid reflux. Unfortunately, these medicines left her feeling nauseous and without appetite, and she began to lose weight. A pediatric gastroenterologist diagnosed gastritis and another medication was added. She also developed chronic headaches, which she had not had before. When the reflux she initially had, progressed to gastritis her parents decided they had had enough of allopathic medications and that those solutions were not working for her; in fact, each set of prescriptions seemed to give her more symptoms instead of less. Even though she has discontinued the non-steroidal, anti-inflammatory medicines some four months before our visit, her digestive symptoms had persisted.

I took the full constitutional case, finding out about how she experienced her shoulder pain, her gastrointestinal issues and her headaches, what made them better and worse, how she experienced them. We continued through her likes and dislikes, her family and friendship relationships, what she thought of the sixth grade and what other sorts of things she enjoyed. She was a most articulate and direct young lady who was a beloved member of her family and church communities. She excelled at most everything she tried and was a good friend to all. She was acutely sensitive to the feelings of others, especially those of her mother; she seemed mature beyond her years.

I had many other thoughts as I saw this patient, besides needing to assess which homeopathic remedy would best match her presenting state. As many of us have read in the news recently, allopathic medicines are not all tested on children and strong drugs can have serious side effects, especially on sensitive and smaller individuals. When I see a patient who has complaints that seem largely due to orthodox drugs, I wish I would have had the opportunity to offer treatment at the time the initial issue had appeared. Though we cannot turn back time, we can pick up the case wherever it is and start working our way through.

With regard to a constitutional homeopathic remedy for Laila, my differential diagnosis, supported by my repertorization, revealed the remedies *Phosphorus, Pulsatilla* and *Carsinosinum,* the latter of which I settled on, based on my understanding of that remedy. I prescribed *Carsinosinum* 200c, one dose taken in the office.

I also wanted to use some tried and true naturopathic approaches to help heal some of the tissue damage in the gastrointestinal tract, due to anti-inflammatory medication. The botanical treatment approach is one that focuses more on stimulating proper digestion, while coating and supporting the mucus membrane lining of the esophagus and stomach. For patients such as this, both children and adults, I recommend a product called DGL, or deglycerinated glycerrhiza. This works to help sooth, nourish and support healthy mucous membrane lining of the esophagus, stomach and intestine. It comes in different flavors, the tablets are chewed before a meal and most can tolerate the taste. We also use Slippery Elm lozenges to help soothe the lining of the gastrointestinal tracts. I encouraged them to try some teas such as those containing slippery elm and marshmallow or a product called Throat Coat (also good for sore throat!) tea by a company called Traditional Medicinals. All work at soothing and supporting the lining as described above.

As far as lifestyle adjustments, I recommended drinking as little as possible, to nothing, *with* meals but to drink water freely between meals. I encouraged Laila to chew her food well and slowly to give her food a bit of a head start with the digestive enzymes present in her saliva. I suggested that her largest meal be at lunch time or in the late afternoon and that the best thing for her to do after eating was to have a short walk or at least be able to sit tall, as opposed to lying down. We also spoke about the importance of sticking with all the things that helped keep stress down like playing with her friends, bicycling, dancing, reading, talking!

I saw her 6 weeks later when she and her mother reported that the gastrointestinal system was much improved. She had many more days now without stomachache or reflux. She no longer complained of headaches and she felt much better over all. Her shoulder however was still bothering her.

We waited with the remedy and modified some of the other items she was taking with an eye to discontinuing them when they were no longer necessary.

Some might wonder, why not just give the remedy. In a case like this, where there has been clear tissue damage, I like to do what I can to help build up and renourish the area. These other, non-toxic, effective and not habit forming approaches, which do not have side effects, are an elegant balance with constitutional homeopathy. Would she have gotten better without them? Perhaps, but perhaps not as quickly. She also now has at her fingertips several things she can use at the first sign of any discomfort in the gastrointestinal system.

Her shoulder continued to bother her for some months. Once the gastritis was better and holding its own for about 4 months, I tried her on a trial of natural anti-inflammatory medications to include Curcumin, which is derived from tumeric and Bromelain, which comes from pineapple, with extra vitamin C. After about six weeks on that protocol, she finally got relief from the shoulder pain. As softball season was fast approaching, this improvement gave her tremendous relief. Thanks to some gentle and effective natural medicines, she is hoping to be a starting softball infielder this spring.

Some Thoughts on Homeopathic Family Practice: Does Parenting Impact Constitutional Types? Should Constitutional Types in Children Impact Parenting?

Visit any local library or bookstore and you will notice an ever-growing section on parenting. The section begins with books on infertility and pregnancy and moves quickly on to problems of nursing and sleep, tantrums, how to handle your difficult toddler, your high-energy child, your spirited child, your clingy child, your artistic child, your genius child, etc. Whatever type of child you are blessed with, there is a book out there to help you navigate the early years!

The best thing about any of these books is the fact that when a parent finds one they can relate to, it makes the parent feel better; they are not such a bad parent after all, other people have a child like 'impossible Johnny', or 'quirky Susie.' In our times, there is little if any family support for the wonderful, if at times impossible, job of parenting. The extended family is almost extinct. With so many single-parent families, or families with two parents working full time or simply the stressed-filled lives so many lead, such books lend emotional support to parents seeking just that.

Homeopathy is one system of complementary medicine which is used to treat both physical and more emotional issues. It is gentle, non-toxic and effective and when applied accurately can go a long way to helping with the large and small issues that arise in the raising of a family. What is the role of the homeopathic practitioner in addressing parenting issues with our patients, or rather with the parents of our patients? Are there things we know as homeopaths about remedy types in children, which could help parents do a better job? What follows are some of my ideas related to these questions and how I handle them in my practice.

I see the children in my practice with their parents until they are about age 7 or 8, then I offer the child the opportunity to see me alone, at least for part of the visit. If there are things the parent wants to tell me that they do not necessarily want to say in front of the child, I will ask the parents to come in first. I particularly like to get the story without the child if the visit is about behavior issues, discipline problems, social problems, school concerns, personality problems, etc. It doesn't feel appropriate to talk about those issues in front of a child, right off the bat.

I will bring the behavior issues to light later, when I am alone with the child, but at least this way, I will have some context for the discussion and case taking. I may also bring up the subject with the parent and child together, to see the reaction and interaction within the family, to look at the language use, the ability to communicate and the emotional issues which arise.

When I am finished getting the story of the child, I may have some thoughts about what I've seen or not seen in the interaction between the parent and child. Generally speaking, I keep these observations to myself, perhaps use them in my homeopathic analysis. That is, if I see a dictatorial child who contradicts everything the mother says, belittles the mother in front of me, I'm thinking about homeopathic remedies like *Lycopodium* or *Anacardium*—depending on the presenting issues and other confirmatory symptoms. A passive dependent child, who constantly looks to the parent for support and help, can't make eye contact, who, upon questioning keeps saying to the mother, "I don't know...What do you think, Mommy?" probably needs a remedy like *Pulsatilla* or *Staphysagria*, regardless of what the chief complaint is.

Whatever my personal assessment might be, there are many ways to parent. And certainly as a practitioner of homeopathy, we have a wide range of what we consider 'normal'. Like the correctly chosen remedy, given based on the individualizing characteristics of the child, children need different things from their parents, even within the same family. So if problems seem glaring, I assess the situation to see if the parent is open to suggestions. And if so, I offer gentle suggestions about setting limits, or using 'I' statements, finding more childcare, less childcare, the use of behavior modification or suggestions for encouraging responsibility. Sometime I ask the parents if they have areas of special concern or questions or things they want to discuss beyond what they brought the child in for, anything that relates to how they parent that particular child. There is often appreciation on the part of the parent to have a place where these issues can be raised and talked about, even if briefly.

What other kind of advice do I give parents? Sometimes it is specific and related to the constitutional type of the child. If I see a *Calcarea carbonica* child giving the parents a very hard time with every transition, I remind the parents about giving this type child the 10 minute warning when they will need to leave, then the 5 minute warning, then the two minute warning, and then depending on the child's age, helping them get the shoes on if necessary. I explain that by describing what is going to happen and narrating as it is happening and then positively reinforcing it, once it has happened (i.e., 'You really did a great job getting your coat on and helping us get out the door on time,') you can greatly increase the child's cooperation about making these everyday necessary transitions.

The *Calcarea carbonica* child may have terrible fears and anxieties and perhaps even nightmares if they see frightening images on television or at the movies. I am not sure it is a bad thing to be sensitive to such visions, especially for the very young, so I encourage most of my patients to avoid this exposure if at all possible. Children learn best by doing, not by watching. The television has become the great All-American babysitter, not necessarily to the benefit of children.

Kids who need the remedy, *Stramonium* will also have horrible fears after seeing scary things, whether on television or in pictures in books. I once saw a little *Stramonium* girl, brought in for recurrent urinary tract infections and nightmares. Seemingly innocent videos would send her screaming in fear. The one the father described was *Winnie the Pooh,* the episode where Pooh gets stuck in Rabbit's doorway and while there, Rabbit draws a black, crooked and frightening smile on Pooh's bottom. At least that's how this little girl perceived it. This otherwise benign and gentle movie caused increasing anxiety for the child; the stress and fear mounted exponentially as it moved toward that scene, that the father finally learned to fast forward past that part, while the child grew increasingly agitated throughout. She would be sure to have a nightmare that night. It does not matter that most children find this a delightful and sweet story. It does matter that her predisposition towards needing *Stramonium* led her to feel fear and anxiety. Parents need to screen what these kids see and if they are in a phase of nightmares and heightened fears, it is best to help them avoid such encounters altogether while the remedy is working on shifting their predisposition away from this sensitivity.

For the *Tuberculinum* child, who might be very difficult for the parent, I always recommend that the parent or caretaker get the child out of the house at least a few times a day, weather permitting. They have a strong need to go 'bye-bye.' Even babies and toddlers already have that desire to travel. They need a change of scenery – it doesn't really matter where – the library, park, shopping. Some parents think it is the gentle rocking motion of the car, but for these kids it is really the change of scenery which makes them better.

For an older *Pulsatilla* child who has deep and constant need for attention and affection, I will often suggest that the child be given something of his or her own to take care of, a guinea pig, or hamster, provided the mother herself does not have excessive fear of rodents! In so doing, we take a child with excessive need and let her shower a pet with loads of love and affection, which seems to help the whole family dynamic.

If I see a painfully shy child, who needs *Silicea* or *Staphysagria*, I keep my voice very low in the interview. I match their demeanor as best I can. These are the children who need very little discipline and if I see either parent overly disciplining this child for a small infraction (biting the nails, splitting hairs, not sitting up straight), after the child has left the room and if the parent seems open to it, I will explain a bit about the remedy and how this type of child generally doesn't need a lot of harshness to come round right away. Of course, with the case of many a *Staphysagria* child, it is a great possibility that they became a *Staphysagria* child because of a harsh, loud, sometimes violent parent.

What about the fact that the homeopathic remedy can help with these more temperamental issues? It will. And it may also take time. Parenting support can help the remedy work faster by removing some of the irritants to that child's day. The child can put more energy into attaining balance if there is less constant conflict, unnecessary discipline or emotional turmoil. It's like a bit of prevention, if you will, on the part of the parent. And most parents who live with a tantrumming toddler, emotionally needy kid, or difficult adolescent, will be just as happy to put in a bit of effort to head off trouble, if possible.

Of course, this can be taken to the extreme. Many parents with challenging children of all ages have developed elaborate and wide-reaching strategies of avoidance. 'What can I do to avoid a situation which will set Sarah off?' Or, 'How can we plan this day so as to keep Steven in a good mood?' There is nothing by definition wrong with trying to create a peaceful environment and trying to initiate pleasant events, but parents' energies and resources can be severely taxed from the constant micromanaging of a child's life. It can also have a negative impact on the rest of the family. Thankfully, we do see that the right remedies, in addition to some support in parenting, can shift the balance in the child, and then in the family, back to a healthier place.

In families where there are many children or a number of children spaced very closely, and every child suffers from lack of attention, I encourage the parents to try to set up some time each week or month which is 'special time' for one of the parents and the child in question (ideally for each child). The children really look forward to this and enjoy it. It gives time for the parent to get to know the child, away from the bustling family, outside the usual roles they fall into, within the family. A usually rambunctious child can become sweet and affectionate, jabbering on about this and that. A usually bubbly and spacey child can become quiet and calm when alone with the parent. This activity is a rare, inexpensive and meaningful treat that family members can give to each other.

What about the terribly over-attached child who is nursing at four, in a family that is doing the 'family bed?' I have seen many families where this is the situation and it seems to be working fine for everyone. Wonderful. There are other families who do not fare as well. The most frequent problems encountered in my practice by these families, in terms of what brings them into the homeopath are: asthma, behavior problems, difficult toilet training, early tooth decay, ear infections and severe separation anxiety. What I find is that with the correct remedy, the child will often decide to stop nursing and will show that they want their own bed. I have also seen *many* toddlers and preschoolers in happy nursing relationships with their mothers. As the physical symptoms begin to decrease – less asthma, or fewer, less severe ear infections – many of the other power struggles seem to also fade. In these situations, it can be quite helpful to treat mom simultaneously.

What about when I see a child whose parents are having obvious relationship problems, difficult communication, conflict about reporting symptoms or agreeing about health care choices? I do the best I can to take the case. If that relationship is so negative as to make the case taking difficult, I have the child leave the room, if they are old enough, and try to honestly reflect what I see: a child caught between fighting parents, or a child anxious because of the parents' conflict. I try to focus these observations on the child, as s/he is the patient at hand. I make frequent referrals to family therapists in our area and see the remedies as essential partners to that therapy work.

As to the disruptive or violent children who come into my office, I will let things run their course for a time, mostly to see how the child 'does their thing' and to see how the parents handle it. I can get a lot of information about the remedy by sitting back and taking it all in. I will often come on heavy at some point. 'Hey, those are my toys, you may not throw them at your brother,' in a somewhat raised voice. Some kids back right down and retreat to the mother's lap - perhaps a mischievous child needing the remedy, *Sulphur*. Others feel egged on by this reprimand and carry on with gusto, as in the case of patient needing the homeopathic remedy *Medorrhinum*. I am not being mean, just seeing how certain stimuli will impact a patient. I set clear rules and stick to them. I set the limits if the parents don't, though I defer to them initially.

I have had some truly unbelievable experiences with little patients. One time I went out to get a four year old child who was brought in for ADD. I always question that diagnosis for that age child, so was curious when I looked at this intake form. Before I could extend my hand to greet the child's mother, he lunged at me and before I knew what hit, had his chompers squarely sunk into my bottom. Not one to be easily ruffled, I asked the mother, 'Does he greet everyone like this?' I think it was most shocking to my receptionist, who just sat there, phone dangling, jaw dropped, as I excused myself to the ladies room to regard my garments. (He did very well over the course of a number of years on the remedy *Tuberculinum*!)

I have been poked, prodded, pinched and spat upon (not all in the same day, I'm happy to report!) Parents feel horrible when their child does something like this, and I certainly don't feel great, but I try to assure the parents that it's better for me to see their child in action, to find the right remedy and help them move beyond that point. If there are episodic types of illnesses like tics or seizures, tantrums, or other behaviors that the parents feel I should see, I will sometimes ask them to video such an event and send it to me. Pictures can paint a thousand words.

As to all those parenting books, I would like to recommend some very helpful ones. Firstly, for the totally overwhelmed, especially first-time mother, who has an intractable case of 'milk brain' and feels that her mind went out with the placenta,

I prescribe *Operating Instructions* by Anne Lamott (Fawcett, 1996) a sometimes hysterical, always thought-provoking journal of the first year of that first time mother's life with her son. Also essential to laugh away the (mild) post-partum blues is the comic book *Baby Blues, This is Going to be Tougher than We Thought*, by Rick Kerkman (Contemporary Books, 1991) which has left more than one new parent tear-struck with laughter. When communication seems to be the biggest problem for any age parent/child, the best practical book which offers immediate results is the classic, *How to Talk So Kids Will Listen and Listen So Kids Will Talk* by Adele Farber and Elaine Mazlich (Avon Press, 1980). (Some years ago I found not one, not two, but three copies of this book on my bookshelves. I pick up spare copies at tag sales or used bookstores to give to friends and patients. When my daughter, then eight years old and already an avid reader saw it, she opened it up. She started reading choice sections of comic strip renditions of 'before and after' scenarios of communication problems resolved, out loud to her then 5 and 6 year old brothers. They sat there aghast. 'Mommy and Daddy studied this stuff-wow!')

Topics as described in the table of contents include: How to Help Children Deal with their Feelings, Engaging Cooperation, Alternatives to Punishment, Encouraging Autonomy, and Freeing Children from Playing Roles. It's inexpensive, an easy read and has a very big 'oh, yeah!' factor. It seems so simple, how come I didn't think of it? I urge most parents in need of a little direction to read it. There are so few requirements for being a parent and there has been so much bad parenting out there. Taking time to learn some basic techniques and skills can help immeasurably.

If the main problem is sibling rivalry, the most complete

and usable book is also by Farber and Mazlich: *Siblings Without Rivalry*. (Avon, 1988). This book has changed the lives of many families with more than one child. It is direct and easy to pick up on their suggestions. More than anything it gives parents strategies to address the sometimes difficult and frustrating situation of children who constantly bicker, fight or threaten each other.

If I see a situation where the parents are clearly unable to set age appropriate limits on their child, especially toddlers and preschoolers, I may suggest the book *1-2-3 Magic*, by Thomas W. Phelan, PhD (Child Management, Inc., 1995) which is a bit harsh in its philosophy but models a very effective way of giving time outs. It's not for everyone's taste, and that technique is not appropriate for every child, but it can be very effective for the kids who push every limit to the max.

Treating children and their families with homeopathy has been a challenging and rewarding experience for me over the last twenty years and I know that a well-prescribed homeopathic remedy can shift the family dynamics in good and unexpected ways.

House Calls

Once during a long cold winter, I had the opportunity to pay a house call to a very sick child. I was reminded about the wonderful art of medicine, in which going into a patient's home can offer abundant and useful information (what and how they drink or don't, how they lie, how many blankets they use, how they respond to attention and affection, what it smells like in the sick room, etc.). I felt like a sponge, soaking up symptoms in the room around me in a way which sometimes is less palpable in an office setting with the chronically ill people I more commonly see. But it reminded me that many observable symptoms are also present in the consulting room, if only we remember to feel, look, and perceive.

Randy, a young boy of 6 was crying softly when I entered the room, saying his neck hurt and he felt just awful. A quick review of the case revealed: a high fever, huge swollen glands, bleary eyes, and a flushed face. The acute illness had come on suddenly after he received a number of nasty notes from a classmate at school. He came home crying and carrying on. He was lying with his feet and legs uncovered and with the flats of his hands against the wall. When I asked him why he was doing that (because I never take any observation at face value, I try to let my observations inform the questions I ask and to then understand what I have seen in a larger context of the person at that point in time,) he replied that the wall was cool and it felt good to him. He had parched lips. His head was in his mother's lap as she gently stroked his hair. His father and sister were nearby watching quietly and not making a peep.

I gave him the homeopathic remedy, *Pulsatilla* 30c. He was in a grief state over being insulted and was feeling forsaken by this classmate. He was warm, thirstless, dry and weepy—all classic *Pulsatilla* symptoms, a prescription most would have found easily.

I also enjoyed preparing a castor oil pack for his neck and reading to both children a favorite book I keep in my doctor's bag, *Goodnight Moon*.

He awoke the next morning without a fever, feeling much more himself. The glands took a few days to go down, but the parents were pleased to see the fever and his sadness gone. I always enjoy making a house call and parents certainly appreciate it!

Special Children, Special Care

The very first time I treated a special needs child was my second week of practice. Ten year old Michael was brought in by his mother, who had a long line of her children in tow. They streamed in, stair-step, 5 others, if memory serves me well. She carried Michael lovingly; caressing his head as she juggled the crew. I assumed he had fallen asleep *en route* and that was why she was carrying him. He seemed a bit big for being held like that, but I was not yet a mother and did not know the ropes! As it turned out, that was Michael, that reflected the extent of his abilities. He had suffered a massive stroke *in utero* and was born with many issues from epilepsy to hydrocephalus to mental retardation. At the time of that first visit his mother also told me that he was blind and deaf, was nourished through a feeding tube, suffering from grand mal seizures and was 'filled to the gills' with mucus. He had an offensive smell to his skin and a vacant expression on his face. His mother wanted help with his seizures and the excessive mucus which sometimes interfered with his ability to breath.

As a young, relatively inexperienced practitioner, I was a bit taken aback. I was taken aback by many things: the sheer number of his issues, the intensity of his symptoms and the degree to which his life seemed to hold so very little promise. But equally as impressive to me was the burning love his mother showered on him and how each of his younger siblings stood at various times during the office visit and rubbed an arm or a foot or cooed at him. His mom, a saint in any regard, was patient and strong and single minded. She wanted help for Michael and heard I could offer it; she didn't much care what I would recommend, she wanted the full treatment.

I remember excusing myself at one point, scurrying back to our break area, just sitting down and taking some deep breaths, that is how overwhelmed I was by this young boy's condition. And realistically, what could I expect to offer, how much might a homeopathic remedy help? Might the seizures decrease? Would the mucus diminish? Could changes be made to the nourishment he received? Was there hope for improving his quality of life? What could I say with confidence about what natural medicine might do for such a boy? The mother's clear request and her unwavering belief in my ability to help Michael, gave me the impetus I needed to get back in that room, take a thorough case and get down to work.

What are we to say when someone approaches and wonders if homeopathy and natural medicine might have something to offer their special needs child? What can we tell them, what kinds of expectations should we have, what in addition to homeopathy should we be sure to talk about? What sorts of referral patterns should we establish?

The term special needs spans an ever-widening lexicon of children with particular concerns, from physical ailments to mental health issues, from emotional and behavioral difficulties to developmental, cognitive and chromosomal problems– and any combination thereof. Special needs—patients come in every size, shape, ethnicity and from all cultures and geographic locations. I ran into a nurse friend of mine while preparing to write this piece and she said, well, aren't we *all* special needs in a way? And don't providers of natural medicine, and homeopathy in particular, pride themselves in treating patients based on the idea that each person is unique and special? Don't we believe that treatment plans are made for specific individuals, not diagnoses?

I had to agree. And I know that in addition, approaches to learning, parenting and discipline are best created and executed according to the person being addressed and are best received and most effective when really tailored to the person at hand, based on things like personality, temperament and unique sensitivities. But of course, our world does not always work that way. In homes, in schools, in doctors' offices there is often a one-size-fits-all mentality, which does not always best serve the person in need. So yes, in some ways, we are all special needs but in the context of this article, I am addressing those children who fall outside the typical standards of development, mental and emotional normatives and physical health and therefore present parents, school systems and healthcare providers with additional challenges and additional opportunities to let natural medicine and homeopathy shine.

At the outset I am seeking to help the special needs children and adults in my practice—and this is not different for anyone who comes through my door—to optimize their genetic potential. Therefore it is always important for me to understand what the particular diagnosis is that I am working with and what is considered typical of patients with that diagnosis. I take the information in context and with a grain of salt. I am not wed to it, but I also do not want to ignore some of the statistics. I want my prognosis to be realistic. While I am generally an optimistic person and physician, I also do not want to offer false hope. More on that in a bit.

I am sometimes the care provider that recommends that a child be assessed based on the history the parent provides coupled with my examination and observations in the office. That said, often patients come in with hefty stacks of lab work, neuro-psych evaluations, educational evaluations, individual educational programs, reports from school, lists of pharmaceuticals tried, etc.

A diagnosis itself is sometimes very disheartening to a parent; depending on the situation it might confirm their greatest fear or add immense stress to a family dynamic. For other families a diagnosis is almost a relief, somehow confirming a concern or validating a hunch and then in turn enabling the parents to access important supports from different therapists, treatments, care providers, schools, etc., some at home, some at school, some in medical or therapeutic settings.

An accurate diagnosis can also help parents, teachers and health care providers to set appropriate goals for a child in question whether they are medical, educational, behavioral, physical or social. Diagnosis can often help parents, siblings and peers to better understand a child, to better accept certain behaviors or limitations. I recall a younger brother of an autistic patient of mine who used the phrase, 'That's my brother, he's autistic. He's waaaay smart, but he just can't talk yet,' when at the playground, dispelling some of the other kid's worries and caution. Or a mother with a 9 year old daughter diagnosed with bipolar disorder somehow freed her from at least some of the angst she'd felt when he daughter was unreasonable and hateful. Instead of blaming herself or her parenting skills, she was better able to see those behaviors as part of her child's illness.

One caution about diagnoses: Sometimes a diagnosis is given in order for a physician to prescribe a medication. Perhaps such a pharmaceutical is being used in a therapeutic trial, that is, if this works, then Suzie must have had an anxiety disorder or ADD or what have you. But it is important to remember that many pharmaceuticals, especially psychiatric drugs, are generally *not* tested on children and some kids have poor responses and unpredictable side effects. Though a diagnosis can be helpful and is most often essential, caution against arriving at a diagnosis if it seems driven by the desire to medicate. And this drive is not only by physicians, sometimes parents, feeling desperate will also push for medications and it should be said, that sometimes pharmaceuticals are indicated and work well. But diagnoses in general are helpful and do impact treatment protocols and prognoses.

Early diagnosis also offers the possibility of early intervention especially with regard to developmental delays and behavioral issues. Intervening early can support a child's development and give assistance to families. The preschool years offer an unequaled time when the pace of learning and development is rapid; this is why early intervention can be so powerful. Such early work can also offer benefit to the parents and siblings of a special needs child. Early intervention can help parental attitudes about their role and about their child as well as supplying more accurate information and relevant skills for teaching their child.

When there is a special needs child in a family, in addition to accessing and utilizing supports for that child, I always encourage families in my practice to secure support for parents and siblings as well. More typical brothers and sisters can suffer deeply from feelings of neglect, feelings of being the 'survivor,' or the 'thriver.' Such guilt is a complicated feeling alone and may be coupled with resentment, pity, deep empathy and perhaps feelings of responsibility. Some of these siblings seem to be doing just great, but I encourage my families with special needs kids to at very least offer the more typical child the opportunity for some talk therapy or play therapy as well as regularly scheduled alone time with a parent or other loving adults.

Special needs kids can also put additional stress on relationships and marriages, due to the additional time it takes to care for such kids, the time and mental strain that goes into finding the right health care providers, the special diets and therapies, financial constraints, accessing the most appropriate educational settings, etc. Without tending, any relationship is at risk, but in such situations, I try to talk with parents about the essentiality of making time and space for each other and to avoid the blame game, focusing as much as possible on the positive and concrete steps to take to move things in the best possible directions. I will also bring up the idea of some respite for families if they have a child with extreme special needs. Everyone needs a break and often there are resources available to support such time away.

The Internet has provided support for many parents of special needs kids. Although it can be overwhelming to start out, finding websites and chat rooms where others have experiences with similar children can be very heartening and informative. There are websites for most any diagnosis. Some sites that patients of mine have used and found helpful include:

- National Organization of Rare Disorders – a website that lists many unusual diagnoses and then gives further reference to resources and other websites about the individual illnesses http://www.rarediseases.org/
- Disability Resources on the Internet http://www.disabilityresources.org/
- Autism and PDD Support Network http://www.autism-pdd.net/
- Federation for Children with Special Needs http://fcsn.org/index.php
- Learning Disabilities Association of America http://www.ldanatl.org/
- Children's Disabilities List of Lists. Gives links to many other websites and support groups for parents of kids with specific issues http://www.comeunity.com/disability/speclists.html

In-person support groups can also be helpful for pooling information, sharing stories and being around others going through similar trials and small triumphs. Websites and local newspapers are the best ways to access in-person support groups.

When I think of special needs kids, I am thinking about those with Down syndrome, mental retardation, cerebral palsy, learning disorders, neurological disorders, autism spectrum disorders, chromosomal or genetic issues, chronic physical illnesses and those with emotional problems. Should natural medicine and homeopathy play a role in the treatment of these patients? Absolutely! I take a full case just as I would with any patient. I am trying to figure out what is most limiting to the patient at the time of the visit. I try to understand the person who has the issue, everything I need to know about all of my patients applies here as well. So while I want to understand the chief complaint, I also want to understand temperament, personality, food desires, sleep patterns and thirst. I want to know how the patient gets acute illnesses if they do and what kinds of things frighten them. I may need to get a lot of this information from the parent in terms of such details but I will use my time in the office to observe and interact with the child. How are they with strangers? How is the eye contact? How do they do when a limit is set? How do they interact with the parent(s) or sibling(s) in tow? What is the quality of their skin, hair and teeth? How do they respond to a screening physical exam? How do they nurse or eat or drink in the office? How do they interact with or play with the toys?

I think one of the most important thing for the homeopath when treating a special needs child, is to stay calm and to stay focused on taking the full case, just as you would with any patient. Get all the details of the chief complaint(s), do a complete review of symptoms, ask about physical general symptoms. Do not get thrown off by the gravity of the situation or get overwhelmed by the sheer number of symptoms or issues. Stay clear in your line of questioning and keep bringing parents back to things you need to know to prescribe well. It can be helpful to have time set aside where the patient is not in the room both to speak about things best not said in front of the child but also to have time to get an accurate history and chronology. Having an additional adult who can be with the child in a separate space can be helpful here.

For some of these children, especially those with genetic issues or cerebral palsy, it is not that we are going to reverse these kinds of diagnoses. But we can certainly help. We can help the child to have less acute illnesses, we can help improve digestion, sleep, allergies, the quality of skin. We can help with things like improving the spirits, the mood or the confidence. When the child's system does not have to spend energy on these things, they are freed to focus more on development and learning or on connecting with others and having fun.

For those with more emotional and behavioral issues we can expect remedies, alongside consistent, loving and firm parenting and appropriate school settings, to go a long way in stemming the most challenging behaviors. I try to never work in a vacuum with such families. I want outside objective therapists to help with diagnoses and most importantly to help with follow-up assessments. For children in this group, we may need to go through a number of remedies as the child shifts and makes progress. We may see regression or new emotional characteristics show up that again we look at in context of the whole child.

I have helped many families through tough times with difficult children. I have not always been successful in helping these kids, but I have always been stimulated to try my hardest, by parental patience, resolve and commitment to helping their offspring. I have also had the great pleasure of seeing difficult teenagers evolve into loving, capable and sensitive adults, now, sometimes hard to believe, with children of their own.

Parents of kids on the autistic spectrum and those with Asperger's flock to homeopaths' offices and there is much we can offer. In this case, it is most important to focus on what is *most limiting* to the child at that time. For some it will be inability to connect with others, for others it will be violent outbreaks, for others difficulty in learning self-help skills. It is essential to try to figure out what drives the behaviors – like for any patient- and what makes things better or worse. We cannot treat based on the common symptoms of the diagnosis, rather on how this child uniquely manifests this pathology.

It is important to remember that all children with special needs, especially those who have severe pathology will retain physical general symptoms of some of the more common polycrest remedies (Herscu, Paul. *Stramonium with an Introduction to Analysis Using Cycles and Segments.* Pages 15-25 on the Map of Hierarchy.) So when we see a very violent child with issues of anxiety and depression and violent outbreaks who is also constipated, sweaty and craves eggs, we must understand that though those physical general symptoms point to a remedy like *Calcarea carbonica*, that they likely need a remedy that better covers the more serious and in essence, the more limiting aspects of their behavior. Many homeopaths make mistakes here by not focusing on that which is most limiting to the child at the time of the visit.

For special needs kids that have chronic diseases in the physical realm, depending on the illness and the child, there is often much to offer from total resolution relief to helpful palliation. I have one young woman with chronic debilitating migraine headaches who had missed most of her tenth grade year. Over a number of months and several doses of her constitutional remedy, she was headache free. Another patient, born at a mere 2 pounds 3 ounces who had multiple issues from asthma to pneumothorax to severe constipation at our first visit and then from failure to thrive and developmental delay a year later, is five and a robust kindergartener with a massive vocabulary and gross motor skills to rival anyone. With careful nutrition, a number of carefully prescribed remedies, some botanical medicine, physical, occupational and speech therapy alongside lots of TLC, this special needs kids is now just a special kid.

Another topic I am often approached about is treating special needs kids for the typical childhood illnesses that arise or for their chronic diseases that they may have in addition to the things that might categorize them as special needs. There is no reason not to go ahead and treat as we would the typical colds, earaches, skin rashes, strains and sprains, etc., that are part of childhood. I will use homeopathic remedies, botanical medicine and supplements right along with dietary suggestions, lifestyle modifications and home remedies like hydrotherapy and massage. For those kids with chronic illnesses like eczema, asthma, allergies, etc., I will use the information gleaned in the overall case taking and take these other elements into consideration as I go. We can expect good results in these things with either cessation of the problem or reduced incidences of occurrence or lessened severity.

Personally, I am most interested in following my special needs patients over time. I want to use homeopathy and other natural medicines with and for them as they grow, as they go through teenaged years and into adulthood. I want to help families to optimize whatever the genetic potential is for their child. In the building of such relationships my work remains satisfying and challenging. The challenges shift and families adapt. I recall one of my cerebral palsy patients who had done very well on a remedy, with regard to her development in reading and reading comprehension and in a reduction in upper respiratory tract infections. For some reason, I asked this bright and cheerful twelve year old, who had major issues with communication and limb spasticity, what else would she like help with. She opened her eyes very wide and made the signs for 'I don't want,' and then drew two letters, one on each thigh: C and P. How I wish I could have given her that and more.

Back to our story of Michael: Based on his problems from birth, the downy hair that covered his whole body, his chronic and unrelenting mucus condition and the fact that he had ground his teeth right out of his mouth, led me to prescribe the remedy *Tuberculinum*. I asked his mother to return in one month. Much to my surprise and amazement, Michael did have a tremendous reaction to the remedy. He had a marked reduction in his mucus production. Moreover, his grand mal seizures stopped. He simply did not have any more. And then to his mother's delight, he began to track sounds by moving his head, something he had never done before. In truth, as I was writing down this information, I felt the mother must have been reading into some small thing she had observed, but then as some of the younger kids were playing noisily in the office, true to her words, Michael shifted his neck and his head moved toward the loud sounds. I did not understand what this meant. But I did begin to develop a certain concern. As it turned out, these improvements were the only ones that Michael ever made, though I saw him many times over the course of several years. You can bet I stuck with the *Tuberculinum* in increasing potencies, then repeated in low potency, every which way it could be given. I then moved to other seemingly well-prescribed remedies but alas, homeopathy had stimulated Michael just as much as it was going to do. But his mother was a steadfast believer now and truly thought her son might recover. I envied her faith and alas did have the opportunity to help others in his wonderful family, but never again Michael. He died peacefully a few years later, surrounded by his loving family.

What I learned from Michael was that no matter what the condition, I should use the tools I have and try my hardest. Sometimes we see miracles, but mostly it is a matter of following patients over time and making small gains while the other supports and educational and medical approaches are also working. I learned to be optimistic without giving false hope. I learned to use outside sources for assessment and follow up as well as my own observations. I learned and continue to learn that life is not fair, that bad things happen to good people, that families are amazingly resilient and often go to great depths to secure help and resources for loved ones in need. And of course I am daily made aware of all my many blessings in love and life.

How to Stop the Fighting and Enhance Family Harmony

When couples set out to begin families, it is often with the idea that there will be several children and that these relationships will somehow be lovely. In many cases, this comes true and the friendship and camaraderie among brothers and sisters is formative, supportive and lifelong. Just as often, however, things backfire. Subsequent children born into families wreak havoc with older siblings, and parents find themselves playing referee and arbitrator all day long. As children get older, sometimes patterns in relating shift; but often they do not. Instead they may escalate, and time at home with siblings especially on weekends or summer vacations can be unbearable for all. The screaming, hate-filled arguments, hitting and other aggressive actions complicate and stress family dynamics.

Most parents are at a loss for how to handle such situations—preventively, in the moment of flaring emotions, and after things calm down. Unfortunately, well -meaning parents often make matters worse. Sibling rivalry can be difficult for parents and children alike, especially for those who don't handle discord well. In many families, we see separate televisions and/or computers to keep kids apart. Or we find each person over-scheduled so that time at home together is minimized. But solutions like that deny a family the opportunity to work together, to learn basic communication skills and to gain the ability to work out differences, not to mention having family relationships that are loving and enjoyable. In my experience both as a physician and as a mother who raised three children, I can say without hesitation: There is help, there are solutions to such major family problems, and there is plenty of reason for hope. With correct homeopathic constitutional prescribing along with conscious parenting techniques, especially when begun early and kept up, diabolical sibling rivalry can be transformed. Perhaps not into a peaceful, loving, picture-postcard family, but one where communication and respect are primary and where time together, at least more often than not, can be tolerated or even enjoyed.

When I first met Daisy I was blown away by her charm. At age four, she could talk to anyone. She flashed a gorgeous white smile at my receptionist, offered to help both older and younger kids in the waiting room play area, and gave me a big hug upon being introduced. She was chubby, almost Rubenesque—if you can use that word to describe a preschooler! Her long blond hair, pulled back into a high ponytail, swung behind her like another limb. Her rosy cheeks came to a central point in her red and full lips. She was flirty, confident and amazingly robust.

The chief complaints Daisy's mom had written on her daughter's intake form were: asthma, jealousy, behavior issues and violence. It was difficult for me to reconcile the bright little girl before me with the notion of behavior problems. She seemed so cute, outgoing, helpful, effusive and capable. I had watched her herd together her family's belongings, and like an ant, she seemed to carry more than her own weight as they made their way back to my exam room. Meanwhile, Daisy's seven year old sister Lisa, who was skinny and pale with small features, sat quietly and almost passively at her mother's side, not taking up much space nor manifesting much energy. According to Daisy's mom, problems between Daisy and Lisa started in Daisy's infancy; it seemed that almost as soon as Daisy became aware of her surroundings, she did not want her sister around. When Daisy was nursing, if Lisa, then three, came over to ask her mother a question, Daisy would bat at Lisa and shoo her away. As Daisy got older and more physically able, she would hit or kick her sister. She wanted her mother's attention to be complete and uninterrupted. If her mom would even talk to Lisa across the playroom while Daisy was at the breast, Daisy would clamp down on the nipple and start pummeling her mother. At first, most people thought this was somehow endearing, but Daisy's mother began to worry almost right away. Comparing notes with other parents, she learned that Daisy's behavior was unusual; they told her that their older children were more likely to be jealous of the younger one, not vice versa.

In general, I would agree with this observation. When a child is born into a family, they more or less accept their position. That said, someone with a very strong personality can seemingly come into this life with his or her own agenda. Daisy's was clear: pay attention to me and me only. Funny thing was, she loved her sister and always wanted to play with her; as long as Lisa went along with Daisy's plans, everything went fine.

In addition to the jealousy issue, Daisy hit the terrible twos with force and passion, and she had not outgrown them even with committed parents who set limits and stuck to them. Her parents instituted time-outs right before she turned two—but it didn't seem to work. Daisy was still in time-out frequently each day. She would carry on, complaining and yelling about being put in her room; and after the five minute time-out, she'd go right back at it, arguing about why she'd been put there in the first place. Most of her transgressions were related to hitting, kicking, biting, scratching, or otherwise abusing her older sister. There was a zero tolerance rule in the house for such behavior, yet the frequency of theses events was on the rise. Daisy's mom could count on four to six major temper tantrums a day where this little dynamo would throw herself on the floor, kicking and screaming when she did not get her way. Otherwise, Daisy was incredibly fun loving and easygoing, and once over her outbursts, engaging, helpful, sociable and ready for action. It was difficult for anyone to stay mad at Daisy because of her remarkable charm.

Unfortunately, this was the worst possible kind of sister Lisa could have hoped for. Even though Lisa was several years older, she would usually acquiesce to whatever Daisy wanted. In this way, Lisa would avoid conflict, keep the peace, and in her mind, perhaps, continue to receive her parents' praises. Of course this was terrifically unfair, and Lisa was almost receding into having no self, no desires, no backbone and no grit. (Some years later, I also treated Lisa, who responded well to a homeopathic remedy and began to blossom and assert herself. I wish I had had the opportunity to treat her sooner!)

The report from Daisy's preschool was mostly fine. She was a bit pushy and domineering to the other kids but otherwise helpful and appropriate. A few times she had elbowed or shoved her way to something or someone she wanted, but when reprimanded she seemed to understand that such behavior was not acceptable. Her mother was relieved that at least Daisy's most aberrant behavior had not found its way into the classroom.

Daisy had some asthmatic breathing difficulties especially when the weather was warm and damp. She often had a lot of yellow, green mucus from the nose, had had conjunctivitis several times, also with lots of yellow discharge, and seemed to have postnasal drip that she was unable to cough up. These symptoms were better in the colder months, and in fact, Daisy seemed to prefer wintertime in general. She never wore a hat, and her parents had a hard time getting her to even wear socks in this cold New England climate. She took some medications daily for the asthma and used an inhaler as needed.

Daisy had mild eczema that was also worse in the summer, behind both knees and a bit in the bend of the elbow. Her mom used *Calendula* ointment when the eczema was especially bothersome in the warm months.

Daisy loved food and would eat and drink almost anything. She was fond of sweets and juicy things, fruits and popsicles. She ate with gusto and great appetite. Her mother wondered if she should be curtailing Daisy's food intake, and she worried about Daisy's weight. She wished Lisa would eat half as much.

Daisy slept uncovered always, in the knee-to-chest position. Her mother asked me if it was normal for a little girl to masturbate. I asked what she meant. She said that Daisy would put near anything between her legs and rock back and forth. I told her it was not abnormal, but that if it happened frequently and distracted her from doing other things, or if she did it in preschool or in public, she should be stopped and told that was something best done alone in her room at home.

The remedies that I considered for Daisy were: *Belladonna* and *Lachesis* for her intensity, jealousy, violent outbursts, internal heat and asthma; *Sulphur* for her robustness, extroversion, eczema and asthma; and *Medorrhinum* for her amazing ability to connect with people of all ages, her passionate intensity, her easy slip into and out of aggression, her tendency to masturbate, and her excessive green, yellow mucus discharges. Ultimately, I chose *Medorrhinum* since its indications seemed to best characterize Daisy's symptoms.

When we were finished with the interview, I gave Daisy

one dose of *Medorrhinum* 200c and asked them to return in two months. I also wrote a list of what I wanted to see change:

1. More cooperation
2. Less violent actions towards sister
3. Calmer household
4. Fewer asthmatic symptoms
5. Less masturbation

This was for my purposes but also for her parents, to be sure we were all on the same wavelength in terms of what the remedy was to address. I like writing such a list because then, at our follow-up visit, it gives us a starting point for assessing the efficacy of the remedy. When many of the patient's issues are in the psychological/behavioral realm and I am also suggesting some psychological techniques (more about this later), I like to include some physical elements on the list—things that are much less likely to be impacted by such techniques.

In my experience, the right homeopathic remedy given to key family members can help measurably in situations where sibling rivalry and behavior problems are prominent. Of course, it would be best to treat all the kids involved as well as the parents, but this is not always possible.

Building communication skills -

1. The work of the homeopathic remedy will be strongly supported by conscious effort along with specific parenting and communication skills. I always ask first, to be sure advice is welcome before making any parenting recommendations; for many, this is delicate ground. Daisy's parents were open and welcoming to any help

available, so we spent the better part of the remaining half hour going over some skills that I wanted the mother and father to implement as follows.

Anytime there was an act of aggression toward Lisa, one of her parents was to get in between the girls, put his or her backside to Daisy, and gush concern and care toward Lisa. After that, they would put Daisy in time-out. In this way, they first paid attention (and loving attention at that) to the offended not the offender.

2. When Daisy came out of time-out, they were no longer going to tell her why she was there or engage in any discussion or argument about it. She knew why she had been put in time-out. To bring the subject up again was not needed and, in fact, gave more air time to the child's poor behavior.
3. They were to run, not walk, to the nearest bookstore and buy the two books by Faber and Mazlish: *How to Talk So Kids Will Listen and Listen So Kids Will Talk,* and *Siblings Without Rivalry.* I have used the teachable, logical and compassionate methods offered in those pages with countless families in my practice as well as in my own home. Helping youngsters face and navigate conflict with skill and confidence is a lifelong gift.

The skills recommended in these books will go a long way toward helping families where there is a lot of conflict, but they will not do it all. In situations where the constitutional type or temperament of one or more of the children are not well suited for each other, well-prescribed homeopathic remedies will provide the missing key. I have sometimes been asked whether the changes in parenting strategies could be the main reason behavior issues and sibling rivalry improve in my patients. I answer that while the impact of parenting techniques should not be underestimated, such results show up over time. I have not seen major personality shifts in a month or two just by teaching and modeling communication skills; but I have seen major shifts when a correct homeopathic constitutional remedy was given. The resistant child becomes less resistant, the jealous child less jealous, the aggressive child less aggressive, the passive child more assertive. For many children, the right homeopathic remedy allows the conscious and focused work of parenting to make a difference. And when used together, constitutional homeopathy and parenting skills work synergistically.

Such was certainly the case with Daisy. At our first follow-up appointment, Daisy was her usual exuberant self, but her mother, a reserved and quiet woman, grabbed me in a bear hug in the waiting room. I guess we'd had some success! As it turned out, Daisy was like a new person. All of her good and wonderful attributes had remained, while the abuse of her sister, the intense temper tantrums, and the violent outbursts were nearly gone. Daisy's tantrums were down to once or twice a week and often seemed like pale imitations of her previous displays. Her asthma symptoms had been very good. She had gone several weeks without use of the inhaler—an improvement—though she still had a lot of mucus. Since it was winter then, however, and she tended to improve in winter, the real test of this symptom would come with the warmer weather. Daisy's mother had noticed less masturbating; in fact, she could not recall seeing any in the past two months. In addition, Daisy's eczema seemed to be clearing up. I loved hearing that both Daisy's psychological and physical issues were moving in the right direction. I was confident that the remedy given was correct and that Daisy and her family were still enjoying the benefits of a good homeopathic remedy prescription. So I decided not to give another dose yet but to wait and see how long the benefits of the first dose would last. I asked them to return to see me in three months, but to phone me earlier should the need arise.

Her parents also thanked me for the book suggestions and said they were now buying copies for friends. Though the techniques did not work every time in every situation especially if Daisy or they were very tired or stressed, at least they now felt like they had strategies to use—that is, they had a plan. They were happy to feel less overwhelmed and more directed in how they were raising their girls. This point should be underscored. If parents can feel empowered to be making changes and know they are moving in the right direction, this can help immeasurably. There is nothing worse than not knowing how to proceed. If parents have a plan of action, even if it does not go perfectly each day, at least there is a plan. And if both parents sign on to such a plan, supporting and reinforcing each other, better yet.

Daisy maintained her behavioral and physical improvements over the following year, helped by a few repetitions of *Medorrhinum* at various intervals when it seemed that she needed it. For example, she would get another dose when mild asthma symptoms cropped up in summertime attendant with a slipping back into some of her old behaviors, and she would quickly be back on track.

It's now been four years since Daisy's first appointment,

and her asthma and eczema are problems of the past. Her mom will bring her in now for the occasional acute problem, but Daisy has been mostly well and doing fine in her primary grades. The sibling rivalry has ratcheted way down to the point that the girls get along better and seem to have developed more of a friendly relationship. Their mother talks about overhearing them working out their differences, and she says they do a better job listening to and hearing each other. It's not always harmonious, but it is no longer like non-stop World War III. Daisy has evolved from a self-centered overbearing toddler into an articulate and confident grade schooler, still with a strong will but one that she no longer uses to overpower others. I have not given her another remedy beyond the *Medorrhinum* but imagine at some point she will need *Phosphorus* or *Sulphur*.

Since I first saw Daisy, I have had the opportunity to treat her whole family. Both sister Lisa and mom have done well with the remedy *Carsinosinum*. Without going into great detail about their cases or the indications for the use of *Carsinosinum*, you can think about this remedy as somewhere between *Pulsatilla, Phosphorus* and *Staphysagria*; in other words, a sweet, slightly needy person, who seeks care and protection and cannot tolerate conflict. The dad has done well with *Ignatia*. Like any satisfied customers, Daisy's parents have sent me many patients, those with emotional issues as well as physical problems. Not all of them have seen the dramatic results that Daisy has, but then again, most of them did not present with such dramatic symptoms either!

So, recommend constitutional homeopathy to friends and family who are experiencing a lot of conflict in their lives—along with the Faber and Mazlish books or others on the subject, parenting classes, and communication-building classes. I do not believe that such dynamics and skills learned in families and between siblings stay only in the home. Learning how to be cooperative with others and to listen and speak with openness and respect are essential skills to being a successful person in most any path one might choose, and a family with children is the perfect place to begin. In the *Siblings Without Rivalry* book, a favorite goal of mine is 'finding solutions that everyone can live with.' One time many years ago when my own children were in elementary school, we passed an anti-war rally in our town. My son turned to me and said, 'Ma, I don't think the mothers of the people involved in that war were ever taught how to find solutions that everybody could live with.' In that moment, I knew all our years of working toward family harmony were well worth the effort.

Mother's Day

Mother's Day one year, Paul built me a clothesline. I had one some years back but it had to be taken down to make room for the potting bench we put in off the side of the shed. I have missed early mornings hanging wash to dry. For me, it's meditative and relaxing, pinning up clothes, one piece after the next. I love seeing the clothes swaying in the breeze or standing perfectly still in the noonday sun. It's hard to explain, as some things come out unpleasantly stiff (for example, towels and jeans) and when we do 10 or 12 loads of laundry a week, it's not particularly time efficient. But now the line I have is on a pulley and I can hang wash right from the deck! Feels like I am back to some recent ancestral roots of living in the tenements in the Lower East Side, where I know my grandmother and great aunts hung their wash between buildings and fire escapes to dry in the sooty, noisy air. If family lore serves me right, they probably had a cigarette dangling from the lip while they were hanging off the fire escape just to add that little extra aroma to the clean wash! After that project we took up the next one: to dismantle the kids' swing set. It had become a death trap: all bare wood, splinters galore, rickety and unmoored from the ground. The wood was rotted and disintegrated and the whole unit was an eyesore. We had gotten this set after placing an ad in the paper (before *Freecycle* was born!), and actually got calls for three sets that day. We pawned two others off to friends and kept this one, which we added to from time to time- a new slide, a plank to walk up, the beloved cargo net.

As Paul sawed it into pieces, I looked at the swings lying limply on the ground and the cargo net in a yellow heap. I saw the newly opened grassy part of the yard where the kids had spent so many hours playing, making up games, digging in the nearby sandbox; all these pages in the book of our family, now turned. I remember doing 'underdogs,' where you push the kid from behind all the way up and you run under the swing. Sophie pleading, 'One more, Mommy, one more... pretty pleeeeese.' I remember holding each of them by the little hand as they came down the slide, until they were old enough to climb up and go down themselves. I remember letting a hose run down the slide and putting a little kiddie pool at the bottom, glee of the slip and splash. I remember being unnerved when one of them, probably Misha, at two or so, climbed across the top like a spider up on all fours, me looking out, horrified from the kitchen window and seeing him ten feet up and having a conniption! I remember having endless catches with Jonah while he was swinging, 'throw 'em faster at me, Ma!' I remember making forts with big sheets and tea parties with mudpies underneath. It was the first place I saw the kids doing pull-up and chin ups and it was always the centerpiece of any obstacle course they created. As we are thinking about high school graduations, kids getting driving licenses and new boy/girlfriends and our sons passing the six foot mark on the wall where we have measured them since they could stand..... Paul and I can embrace this next phase of launching these young adults into the world. We are everyday present to how short childhood is, how brief a time it is that we all live under one roof in this family grouping. Making the time together as peaceful and loving as possible was always our goal and we see the fruits of our labor in the wonderful people our children have become, in every accomplishment they have achieved. How difficult those early years were! The constancy of it, the ongoing demands, the calling on deep resources for problem solving, for good spirits, for creativity, for patience. We always said the minutes drag, but the years fly by. Thankfully we were present to it all, we were there much of the time and we experienced these children in all their glory. And how the job of parent helped us to grow and helped us to evolve into better people and better physicians, too.

We all went together on one of our favorite walks recently, along a little river, sitting on a wooden bridge in the sun and just talking, the three kids laying down one head on one lap, another on someone's belly. Sitting there was so peaceful and quiet and happy. The deep sighs felt all around, the easy smiles and erupting laughter, oh, these are images a parent relishes!

SO! Happy Mother's Day and Happy Father's Day, whatever time of the year it is! I hope there are beautiful days and that you have time for reflection and appreciation. And I hope that all the children we love and cherish will go out and live long, healthy and productive lives, filled with love and purpose, adding their own strong voices to this crazy world.

Asperger's Syndrome. What is It? Can Homeopathy Help?

Many homeopaths have had the opportunity to treat patients who fall in the grey areas of diagnoses. With regard to childhood behavioral disorders there is often a fine line between unique personalities and diagnostic criteria. This is certainly the case with Asperger's Syndrome (AS). Though symptoms of this disorder have been around forever, the actual diagnosis was first made official in the DSM IV (Diagnostic and Statistical Manual of the American Psychiatric Association) in 1994. It is not clearly known yet about exact rates of occurrence, male/female ratios (though more boys seem to have it) or the extent of genetic tendency (though these sorts of people do seem to run in families). People with AS are often described as being on the autistic spectrum, though generally high functioning and with either slight mental retardation, average intelligence, or in fact, superior intelligence.

A summary of the diagnostic criteria is printed below. It should be noted that the DSM reference is currently under review, a new one comes out periodically and there is some movement to remove the diagnosis of Asperger's altogether and place it instead within the diagnosis of autism. Many people with Asperger's as well as their parents and advocates do not want to see this happen. Having finally arrived at that diagnosis and receiving helpful services, they do not want to turn back to the clock.

This table as well as other important information about AS can be found in a very useful pamphlet entitled, 'Guidelines for Parents: Assessment, Diagnosis and Intervention of Asperger Syndrome' published by the Learning Disabilities Association of America. (412-341-1515) The pamphlet is authored by Ami Klin PhD and Fred Volkmar MD of the Yale Child Study Center.

DSM IV Definition of Asperger Syndrome (APA 1994)

A. Qualitative impairment in social interaction as manifested by at least two of the following:

    1. Marked impairment in the use of multiple nonverbal behaviors such as eye-to-eye gaze, facial expression, body postures and gestures to regulate social interaction.

    2. Failure to develop peer relationships appropriate to developmental level.

    3. Lack of spontaneous seeking to share enjoyment, interests or achievements with other people.

    4. Lack of social or emotional reciprocity.

B. Restricted repetitive and stereotyped patterns of behavior, interests and activities as manifested by at least one of the following tendencies:

    1. Encompassing preoccupation with one or more stereotyped and restricted patterns of interest that is abnormal either in intensity or focus.

    2. Apparently inflexible adherence to specific, nonfunctional routines or rituals.

    3. Stereotyped and repetitive motor mannerisms.

    4. Persistent preoccupation with parts of objects.

C. The disturbance causes clinically significant impairment in social, occupational or other important areas of functioning.

D. There is no clinically significant delay in language (for example single words used by age two years, communication phrases by age 3 years).

E. There is not clinically significant delay in cognitive development or in the development of age appropriate self-help skills, adaptive behavior (other than in social interaction) and curiosity about the environment in childhood.

F. Criteria are not met for another specific Pervasive Developmental Disorder or Schizophrenia.

Although not specifically mentioned in these criteria, it is often noted and confirmed in practice that most of these patients have significant problems with gross and/or fine motor coordination, as well.

So for these patients, their problems lie more in the arena of interpersonal relationships and the inability to read and respond to social cues. Though most people with AS can speak quite articulately and at a young age, it is often difficult for them to communicate. Very often people with AS find single topics on which to focus, learning everything there is to know about a single topic. They may then move on to other topics. I have seen in practice these interests range from model trains to old time records, from butterflies to antique pocket watches. And though these topics give such individuals great focus it is at the expense of being present in this world.

Many times a parent of a child with AS winds up sitting in front of a homeopath asking for help. I have treated patients with AS who are bought in for unrelated problems: asthma, chronic earaches, a skin or digestive complaint—the whole gamut. But increasingly parents are bringing in children because they hope that homeopathy might make it easier for their child to be in the world and function in a more 'normal' fashion. Most of these kids have lives which are not easy and do not benefit from the usual warmth and attention of loving friends and a supportive peer group because, in actuality, there is very little peer group and such patients have numerous difficulties in the emotional realm.

I have seen homeopathy help tremendously in these cases. Certainly for the physical problems that the patient might have, but also for the actual AS itself. So, I encourage all practitioners to welcome these cases into your practices. Once you help one person with this diagnosis, others will not be far behind because information will get shared. I also believe that we will be seeing more people with AS as the years unfold, largely due to earlier and better diagnostic criteria and partly due to other factors which I believe put children more at risk for neurological conditions, in general. These include but are not limited to toxins in the environment, maternal exposures during pregnancy, and early/frequent and combined childhood vaccinations.

Like many newer diagnoses, we may see this syndrome over diagnosed. Certainly we have all seen patients who have many of these diagnostic criteria but do not have AS. So we need to be careful in our labeling of patients and in particular, with this label. An educational, therapeutic or occupational program must take into account all of the patients' strengths as well as limitations and challenges. Now that we have a working definition and insurance companies recognize this diagnosis, many more services are available to these families.

I have frequently sent patients for neuro-psychiatric evaluations when I am not sure what the problem is. I know the child is not 'normal,' yet I'm not exactly sure what's wrong. That was the situation in the case presented here. Sometimes in practice, the actual specific diagnosis is not critical, but often it impacts my prognosis and rate of prognosis. I like to know what I am working with— are there nutritional components of the problem I should know about; are there genetic elements; what is random and lastly, what are typical allopathic treatments?

I especially want to know this last bit of information. As a homeopath, my highest calling is to heal the sick. If there is an allopathic approach that is effective and does not have serious or long-term side effects, there are times when I might choose that approach first. For some neurological and psychiatric conditions, a patient will do best if they simply can get a break from what it is they're going through. Instead of charging ahead thinking that homeopathy is the best or only way, we need to look at all our options. We can always come back to homeopathy, and often with a bit more clarity and self-understanding the patient can give us a better case, or at least a case which is easier for us to prescribe for. This is not particularly true for AS, unless there is simultaneous severe depression or anxiety.

There are wonderful support services available for individuals and families of folks with AS and I have mentioned a few at the top of page 91. The Internet is a terrific resource, as for most things these days; there is no longer the need for people suffering from this diagnosis or caring for someone who has AS to feel alone.

A Case of Asperger's Syndrome

I saw this eight year old boy first in 1995. The chief complaints are attention deficit disorder and allergies. Even before the interview began, I got quite a bit of information. I try to get a glimpse of my patients while they are sitting in the waiting area, before they know I am watching. Sometimes you can see things that you would otherwise not get a chance to see. On this occasion, I see a plump young boy sitting with headphones on, tapping his fingers on the arms of the chair, swinging his legs, in good rhythm and seemingly happy, albeit in his own world. He is very friendly and polite when I go out to introduce myself; he extends his limp hand for me to shake, though keeps his gaze at the floor. He is listening to classical music. I note that he is dressed in a particular fashion: elastic waist pants, Velcro shoes, Velcro closures on his jacket.

I bring the patient and his parents back to my office. The mother begins with the main complaint. She reports that her son has a constant runny nose, he is pale and frequently has bouts of violent sneezing. If he gets sick he can develop an asthmatic type cough. His younger sister has asthma, too. When he has asthma he is very frightened, feels as if he will die from not being able to breathe. His pediatrician feels he over-reacts—does not feel that his asthma is so bad. They use inhalers to control the asthma. (Right away, I observe the boy is doing a fair amount of winking and blinking and staring off into space. The facial tics initially look like allergic type wrinkling of the nose but I then see that there were many varied types of grimaces. The constant progression of grimaces gives him a bit of a strange appearance; making him look alternately curious......bothered......confused. They are not obviously in response to the interview or conversation going on around him. He did seem to be listening but did not take part in the dialogue. He is restless and fidgety, swinging his legs, and repetitively kicking the chair beneath him. He frequently stares at the ceiling or at a spot on the wall and hums off and on throughout the interview. Though one can never be totally objective in case taking—indeed, in homeopathy we can use some of these subjective feelings and findings to our advantage—I have the feeling that he is a bit odd).

I continue along our line of questioning, asking if there is anything that makes him worse (referring to the asthmatic condition, I thought.) The mother responds that the worse thing for him is choice time. (A forty-five minute period of time at school where the children are able to choose from one of five or six activities—some solitary, some in small groups; it could be an art project, a game, an activity based on a topic being studied, etc.) He cannot handle that lack of structure, having to make open-ended decisions about how to spend his time, and having to relate to the other children.

So the case had taken a different turn, away from what was written on the intake form under Reason for Today's Visit, and onto what was really concerning the mother. When these detours occur it is essential that we go with them, as it is often where the case unfolds. We can always go back and get the details and modalities of the asthma or arthritis or headaches, but often the right time will not present itself again to hear the story the patient wants us to hear. She went on:

He has terrific fear of having a bad dream, he has often suffered with night terrors and bad dreams. He screams and shrieks and is absolutely unable to hear his parents or accept comfort. It terrifies the parents to see him like that, almost possessed. For years, he would not leave his mother when it was time to go to sleep; in fact, she still has to lie down with him for hours in order for him to fall asleep. He sleeps deeply but is quite restless, moving all over the bed, grinding his teeth and often talking incoherently in his sleep. He often awakes agitated, worked up about something, which he is unable to articulate.

Since these fears came up early in the case, I asked of other fears and there were many. He has tremendous fear of going upstairs by himself, huge aversion to deep water, and a strong fear of drowning. He does not like animals much, especially dogs.

I felt that I would need to speak with the mother alone because I could see that she was getting worked up describing some of these things. There were clearly lots of mental and emotional symptoms, but because of the nature of some of those concerns, I felt it better to speak to the mother alone. Yet, I wanted to try to engage the patient some, experience him first hand, in dialogue. I understood that he checked out psychologically a lot and did that especially if these topics were broached, before I sent him out to be with his father in the waiting room, I asked some more basic physical general type questions and then spent some time trying to talk to him about something *he* was interested in.

In the review of systems, he tells me he gets occasional stomachaches and had normal, daily bowel movements. He loves pizza, tacos, dairy, cheese, yogurt, bread and salt. He is very thirsty for cold drinks.

I asked him what he likes to do in his free time. He glazes over and begins speaking in a staccato type fashion—almost machine-like—about his hobby: model trains. His knowledge is encyclopedic, remarkable really. He speaks with little inflection or expressiveness, but with great intelligence. His mother tells me that he has had other interests in the past, like shell collecting. He stays on each topic until he reaches some point and then it's gone. She and her husband feel mixed about it all. It is fascinating but it seems obsessive and when he's full tilt into something it's like a drug. So they like it, because they get a break from his emotional roller coaster behavior (see below), but on the other hand, it does seem to pull him further away from the family, his peer group and people in general.

When I was with the mother alone, I asked her to describe her pregnancy and delivery, both of which were normal. He was a colicky baby, difficult to please. They spent many a night holding him for hours. He seemed afraid to go to sleep; he would often cry out in his sleep, as if afraid. His baby milestones were normal; sat up, smiled, walked on time, spoke early. He was and remains difficult to console.

His threes were horrible: Constant screaming, crying, tantrums, throwing himself on the floor, inconsolable. The slightest things still throw him off though he tantrums less, he is still difficult to please.

I ask if there are other emotional concerns that the mother has. She tells me that he is explosive, screaming at his little sister if she disturbs him. He can break down quickly and with terrific intensity. It is difficult for him to recover from these episodes and he can remain in a funk for hours. This will occur if something does not go his way or if his routine is interrupted.

He does not handle well any transitions whether to something he wants to do or not.

He is afraid of and hates to be alone, yet has no real friends. He doesn't really know how to be with other children. He's better one on one, terrible in a group, doesn't know how to interact. He does not read social cues and often offends other children by being unaware of personal space, by interrupting or ignoring them or by hurting them physically by being out of touch with his own body placement. None of these behaviors are ever intentional his mother stresses, rather are due to his being unaware.

His best friend is his elderly great uncle who lives nearby. His mother reports that the uncle is very similar to this patient. They share a passion for model train sets and in fact spend many hours researching, shopping for and building elaborate set-ups.

He can be verbally incoherent, has a very fertile imagination especially about trains, but integrated into that fantasy world is quite a bit of accurate information. Television relaxes him, he can space out for hours in front of the television.

He had an early diagnosis of obsessive/compulsive disorder which the parents did not agree with. He is uncoordinated and has difficulty with both gross and fine motor coordination. This is why we see him, at age nine wearing only clothing that does not require buttoning, snapping, zipping or tying. His handwriting is terrible and he has never learned to ride a bicycle. He has taken to doing some writing on the computer which the school and family feel mixed about. If he abandons the writing, it will never get any better, yet the poor handwriting prevents him from further being able to communicate. He will not attempt any new physical activities and shows great fear and discomfort when asked. He has upper body weakness and can be found doing most of his activities lying on his abdomen on the floor holding his head up with his hand. He receives special education in an integrated classroom at school, as well as physical and occupational therapy. His therapy is geared at helping with age appropriate social skills, communication, and strengthening his upper body.

He is very sensitive to high pitched sounds and strong smells as well as the types of materials he wears—it can only be the softest cotton with no tags left to irritate the back of his neck or the waistband area. Gloves and mittens present a problem because they're either itchy or uncomfortable, too tight or baggy.

The mother feels that she has to micro-manage every second of his day to prevent something from going wrong. Of course, this is impossible. Though I have not treated the mother, I believe she needs *Calcarea carbonica,* she really goes the extra mile to organize and carefully plan out every detail of this child's day in order to try and make things go smoothly.

He picks up conversations from three hours or three days ago without regard. It is as if he never stopped talking that first time. He does not read other peoples facial expressions or responses; he speaks in a strange, monotone, inexpressive voice. There is small laughter, almost snickering thrown in here and there, in and out of context. The mother constantly uses the phrase, 'Look at me,' when speaking to him, because he does not like to make, and simply cannot sustain eye contact. Without making eye contact and facing other people when he speaks, it is difficult for him to have real communicative conversations.

If very angry about something, he will hit himself repeatedly, especially on the head. And although he has a fascination with it, he is very afraid of and hates all violence whether in books, movies or music.

That was the information I gathered by listening, by asking and by observing this child. This interview took a little more than an hour. I referred this child to a local behavioral pediatrician for a diagnostic workup. The stress and constant vigilance with which the parents needed to operate made me feel that there really was something diagnosable going on with this child. Indeed, the diagnosis was AS, which though a shock to the parents, helped them to understand what they had been living with all these years. The diagnosis also enabled the family to receive further support services through their local public school district.

He has received *Tuberculinum* and *Calcarea carbonica* from another homeopath without effect. *Pulsatilla* has helped his physical symptoms but made his mental/emotional and neurological symptoms worse.

So the case analysis. When I am taking the case, I want to be sure I end the case having gathered certain information. I want to end the interview *knowing* what it is that needs to be cured. I need to know what I am trying to help. If I don't get that, then all the case analysis, all the computer programs in the world will not help; it's simply garbage in/garbage out. If I realize after an interview that I have six or eight or ten pages of notes, but no real clear understanding of what I'm trying to cure, I know I'm in trouble. This happens to all of us.

We get caught up in the data and leave the patient behind. Or we take the case and lots of beautiful keynotes pop out and we start to see the stars of a constellation and maybe we know that constellation and it feels like we can prescribe based on that pattern recognition. But actually, it's just a string of keynotes and *lots* of people have keynotes of this remedy and that remedy! Turns out, even with all those keynotes in hand, we don't really know what the underlying problem is which needs to be addressed! If that happens, I either need to have the patient come back in, or I need to get them (or the parent in some cases) on the phone and figure it out.

I can pretty much guarantee, that pouring over your notes and rereading all the information that you've written down, will not necessarily help if you don't understand and or have a clear feeling or sense of what the real pathology of the patient is.

If I have that, I can pretty much use any number of approaches and get in the ballpark of a remedy which will help. Once I do have that, I want to see the patient's chief complaint(s) in context of the rest of their life; in essence, I want to know what it's like to be that person, how they go day-by-day navigating all of life's complexities.

If possible during the interview, I try to keep all the information organized. I use Paul Herscu's approach of *Cycles and Segments* to help me keep things in order and to help me organize what is usually lots of detailed information. I try to see the patient's pattern of pathology—how they have the same symptom occurring over and over again in different parts of the body, and also on different levels. For instance, if I have a patient with severe menstrual cramps and frequent constrictive migraines, I would see these as different expressions of the same pathology. I would put these in one Segment. I would then not be surprised to find out that this patient was miserly, cheap and stingy with emotions *and* money. The whole person is cramped and pinched. This is the ultimate in a holistic way of seeing patients.

When we study *materia medica* we can see the same themes running through remedies. If we have a *Medorrhinum* patient with a lot of excess we would expect there to be growths, discharges, passion, temper. By understanding the themes that run through remedies and by looking for the similarities that run through patients outward problems, we can get a clearer view of the patient and not get as easily overwhelmed by too much information.

So, if I can organize my information during the interview, I do. This will help inform my case taking as well. If I have a clear Segment that I understand with a few symptoms in it, perhaps written in rubric form, but not necessarily, then I will try to see what those symptoms lead the patient to do. That will automatically give me the next Segment. I will also try to see what leads the patient to the symptom in question in the first place, that will automatically give me the preceding Segment.

In every patient we also find some symptoms which are opposite to the chief complaint. If we have three or four Segments and we can't see how they are related, I often ask directly about symptoms which are opposite to the chief complaint. For instance, in this case we see the violent outbursts and opposite that, we see the terrific closing off. I will ask this question directly, because I know these opposite symptoms will be there; they may not be as strong as the chief complaint, but they are there.

The beauty in this is that once I have a Cycle completed, if I can do this during the case taking, then I know I am actually done taking the case. I'm finished. Everything else the patient can say will fall into one of these Segments and will make sense in terms of the Cycle of pathology of the patient. This is a great relief to the prescriber! People often talk about the gut pleasing feeling of knowing the remedy, but what if you never feel that? Once I have created a Cycle made up of Segments, I will often feed it back to patient, see if I'm on the right track. They will offer up various corrections or affirmations to what I present, which further helps me to correct my perceptions.

If I can't see how to organize the information *during* the case taking—because the information is flying out at me at a rapid rate, or I'm needing to put a lot of energy into connecting with the patient or perhaps *I just don't see it*, then I take it all home and sort it out there. Mind you, I will still want to leave the interview with the first thing mentioned—*an understanding of what needs to be cured*. But if I have not organized and categorized my symptoms into Segments or a Cycle, that's okay, I'll just see the handful of main problems as separate entities for the time being.

So, with this case, I was organizing the information as it was coming in. Instead of listing all the possible symptoms or rubrics in a laundry list like fashion, I was organizing the symptoms in to a handful of categories, i.e., Segments. I saw the following Segments:

He has a terrific **fear of death** – all of his fears stemmed from a fear of death. This is reflected in: a fear of going to sleep, fear of water, fear of nightmares, fear of suffocation, fear of dogs, fear of being alone and fear of violence.

There is **an element of violence**. Things that fall into this category include the night terrors, grinding of the teeth, hitting himself, screaming at his sister, kicking the chair, restlessness in sleep and grimacing. The grimacing is an uncontrollable bit of energy that comes out in small violent movements.

We can also see **a closed off element** in his introversion, desire to be alone even when with people, obsessive tendency, hyperfocus, (shuts out all other stimuli), difficulty making or maintaining eye contact and expressionless speech.

This set of symptoms can lead to **total self-isolation** where he introverts completely and spends hours and hours in his own world.

He also has **confusion about where he is in this world** manifested when he needs to relate to others, not being sure how to converse effectively, or when he picks up strands of conversations from previous days. He is confused in unfamiliar places, he cannot be interrupted, he is totally lost when in the throes of a night terror.

As these segments made themselves clear, it began to look like Segments of a Cycle I knew—*Stramonium*. But there are many other remedies which share Segments. For instance, *Cuprum* has tremendous violent tendencies—grimacing, grinding the teeth. *Baryta carbonica* has much of the closed off Segment, the inability to make eye contact and the introversion. By looking at only a hand full of keynotes or by focusing too intently on one Segment, we can often miss the right remedy. By understanding the whole Cycle of the patient, how their pathology repeats itself in a consistent, predictable way throughout the individual, we are more likely to get within a handful of remedies—one of which will be effective, early on.

Once we have a few clear Segments we try to see how the Segments relate to each other, what leads from one Segment to another. We can pull together rubrics within each Segment—some large, some small so we do not lose remedies in the repertorization process.

For a fuller and more in-depth discussion on the philosophy behind Cycles and Segments see Paul Herscu's *Stramonium with an Introduction to Analysis Using Cycles and Segments.* For a more detailed, practical hands-on, step-by-step explanation of this approach, see *The Herscu Letter,* which is a twice-monthly e-mail, problem based learning series available through the New England School of Homeopathy.

So I prescribed *Stramonium* 200c. When they came back 2 months later, the mother reported that he had had a good report from school, he was interacting more with the other children and his asthma seems to have stopped. He still had a runny nose. He seemed more easy going to the mother, less in his own world, more in theirs. Transitions were not so difficult. He was making progress academically and in his various therapies.

I have worked with him consistently over the last five years and he has had *Stramonium* a total of five times in different potencies. He was given the remedy *Cannibis indica* once a few years back when the closed off/spaced out part of him seemed to dominate, but it did not have a good effect and going back to the *Stramonium* in a higher potency helped again.

I have been amazed at how he has done. He can now make and maintain eye contact. He relates to both adults and peers in a more appropriate manner. His physical and occupational therapies have been discontinued. He still has his intense interests and remains somewhat obsessive about them. But he has found a number of like-minded friends to pal around with and no longer tantrums. His parents do wonder about the AS diagnosis at this point, as do I. He is still a bit odd, quite intense, but—let's face it—there are many odd and intense people out there!

Is he at risk for other psychological problems as the years go by? I'm not sure but I hope to continue treating him over the years to help smooth the transitional adolescent years with homeopathy.

I wanted to share with you a list of rubrics from the mind section that are often used with this population. Many symptoms will individualize your patient and are not listed here, but here are some of the more general symptoms which may apply to patients with the diagnosis of Asperger's Syndrome:

Absent minded	Approached (by persons being) aversion to
Absorbed	Asking for nothing
Abusive	Awkward
Ailments from (specific subrubrics as apply)	Biting (specific subrubrics as apply)
Anger (specific subrubrics as apply)	Breaking things
Answering (specific subrubrics as apply)	Capriciousness
Anxiety (specific subrubrics as apply)	Cautious
	Childish

Company (specific subrubrics as apply)	Injuring himself
Concentration (specific subrubrics as apply)	Looked at, cannot bear to be
Consolation Aggravates	Mistakes making (specific subrubrics as apply)
Contradiction Aggravates	Music (specific subrubrics as apply)
Conversation, aversion to	Occupation Ameliorates
Discontented (specific subrubrics as apply)	Perseverance
Disturbed (averse to being)	Petulant
Dullness (specific subrubrics as apply)	Queer (specific subrubrics as apply)
Eccentricity	Rage (specific subrubrics as apply)
Fancies (specific subrubrics as apply)	Rocking
Gestures (specific subrubrics as apply)	Selfishness
Grimaces	Senses (specific subrubrics as apply)
Idiocy	Sensitive (specific subrubrics as apply)
Impatience	Shrieking (specific subrubrics as apply)
Impetuous	Slowness (specific subrubrics as apply)
Inconsolable	Spaced out feeling
Indifference (specific subrubrics as apply)	Speech (specific subrubrics as apply)
Industrious	

Spoken to; being, aversion	Timidity
Staring	Trifles seem important
Striking	Unobserving
Thinking (specific subrubrics as apply)	Unsympathetic
Thoughts (specific subrubrics as apply)	

Not all of the patients that Paul and I have treated with this diagnosis have done as well as this child, but without exception, each one has been helped. So along with other problems on this spectrum such as autism and pervasive developmental delay, there seems to be an important role for homeopathy. I hope this has been helpful and that other homeopaths will share their experiences treating patients with AS.

The Homeopathic Treatment of Autistic Spectrum Disorder

Families with members on the autistic spectrum seek homeopathic care for many reasons. Some families seek help because they have always used natural medicine for their health concerns and so this fits into a philosophical paradigm which is consistent with the family. Some feel they are making progress with the programs they have put together for their family member but now a physical plane issue is getting in the way of the progress of treating the autism. For instance, a child who gets frequent upper respiratory tract problems which lead to asthma; each time the child becomes ill, he or she may lose ground in the sphere of communication. So, the homeopath is looked to in order help prevent and treat such infections and illnesses.

Some find themselves in our offices because they are dissatisfied with drug treatments which have been attempted for certain elements of their child's condition; be it attention deficit or obsessive compulsive disorder or anxiety. The medication for this sensitive child, isn't working, isn't working well enough or is causing side effects which are deemed unacceptable. Some have come to us in desperation. Nothing else is working including changes in the diet, nutritional or botanical supplements, working various behavioral and educational approaches and their loved one is still locked up in their own world or perhaps has become violent.

By and large, most of the people that we see for the treatment of autism have been referred by someone else who has had some success using homeopathy. This word of mouth, underscored and amplified by the Internet has led many patients to our office. We are repeatedly amazed and inspired by the tireless efforts of parents on behalf of their children to seek out and secure help and support.

Homeopathic medicines are quite safe: They are known to be non-allergenic, non-toxic and free of side effects. They are prepared from herbal, mineral and animal substances by homeopathic pharmacies, under strict guidelines established by the FDA. Those practicing homeopathy include naturopathic physicians, medical doctors, chiropractors, osteopathic physicians, as well as trained professional homeopaths.

The in-depth interview process delves deeply into the patient's physical, mental and emotional nature. The remedy is chosen by the practitioner after an interview and analysis.

Classical homeopathy, such as that practiced in my office, encourages the prescriber to offer only one remedy at a time.

My husband, Paul Herscu ND and I have worked with many autistic patients, from those with Asperger's Syndrome to those who are profoundly autistic. Most every child has made some improvement, some subtle, others dramatic. A handful have had their diagnoses then questioned. We have had previously mute children begin to speak and those who cannot make eye contact begin to. We have seen many children be better able to learn and interact in social settings, and have watched families begin to enjoy some peaceful times with their children. We have had some resounding failures, like everyone who works with autistic patients; we do seem to help most of our patients and the families we have had the privilege to work with.

Some of these children have been vaccine injured. Others were never vaccinated. We have worked with numerous families where more than one person was diagnosed on the autistic spectrum. There are many routes to autism, many we do not yet know.

Most all of our autistic patients are undergoing other treatments at the same time, from behavioral to nutritional to secretin to chelation and everything in between. Homeopathy does not appear to interfere. It can be difficult to know what is working so we discourage parents from trying something else new when a homeopathic remedy is given.

For first aid and acute conditions which occur in those with autism as well as everyone else, for the vast majority of situations, there are a limited number of homeopathic remedies that would be considered. Remedies that are used over and over again include: *Aconite, Belladonna, Pulsatilla, Chamomilla, Sulphur, Arnica, Mercurius* and *Arsenicum album.* I truly do not know where I would be as a physician and as a mother without these dear friends in the medicine cabinet.

Thankfully, there are wonderful books on acute prescribing, written in a way that enables a parent to choose the correct remedy for things like bee stings, sore throats, teething, and diarrhea. Most of these books will also caution parents as to when it is essential to seek further medical care. No one wants to put a child at risk because of a philosophical belief in natural treatment. There is a time and a place for all types of medicine.

For constitutional prescribing for chronic illness such as autism, I will need to understand all aspects of the child, not just the particular diagnosis, but how the child manifests their problem in all the minute details. This happens in an in-office, in-person interview which lasts for 1-2 hours. I ask questions, make observations and interact with both patient and caregiver. I need to understand little things, like what and how they eat and how they sleep; things related to temperament and personality, like how they behave with new children or changes in routine. I need to understand what will really set them off and what might calm them down. I will be interested in the mother's pregnancy and in the child's earliest months, their development as well as their experience of daycare or school. We try to put the child's illnesses into the context of the rest of their lives and understand them in a complete way. Naturally, I will be observing the relationship between parent and child, how clingy they are, how they respond to limit-setting, how they communicate with each other, or not. For this sort of constitutional care, it is good to have an objective person prescribe (that is not the parent!) and to follow the child over time.

Parents often wonder about the time frame of seeing the effects of a constitutional remedy. We often see influences within that first week, but like to wait at least four to six weeks, before actually assessing the prescribed remedy. This way, we can see patterns and tendencies more clearly while giving the remedy a chance to act. We try to treat children over the course of years as it allows us to address physical, mental and emotional concerns which arise with the various stresses of family life, school, hormones etc. Some of our patients have dramatic results in short order, for others the path is more winding; this has to do with the particular manifestation of the diagnosis, genetic inheritance, other illnesses also present, other treatments being tried, as well as other factors.

There are many licensable practitioners who do homeopathy: MDs, NDs, DOs, NPs — most of whom have studied either on their own or through training programs. There are also professional homeopaths, who do not have an orthodox medical background. It is best to bring your child to someone who has experience treating those with autism. The best source of referral is often word of mouth.

I have always enjoyed treating those people in my practice who present on the autistic spectrum. I suppose it is their individuality, their quirkiness as well as my deep desire to help them and their families. There are no cure-alls for the treatment of autism. However, homeopathy is a gentle, holistic approach which can offer another way to look at and treat these interesting and unique patients.

Chapter 4

For Teenagers

Teenagers, Gotta Love 'Em'

Once when my children were 4, 5 and 7 a woman was watching me at the playground trying to round up my children who were dashing off in three different directions just as we were trying to leave. She said something like, 'Oh honey, you think you have your hands full now, just wait 10 years!' One blessing of several children close in age, is that I seldom had time or leisure to project out that far; it was hard enough getting dinner on the table. As it was, I had good kids who evolved into energetic, engaged and thoughtful teens. But it might not have been that way. I see in my work and in my community, families who have seemingly done most everything right, yet teens have veered into self-destructive behavior, unhealthy relationships, substance abuse, school failure and any other number of things we try to guard against. Then there are those who simply do not engage, do not seem to take responsibility for their lives, who 'fail to launch.' Parents bring in all kinds of teenagers with all kinds of issues for me to treat. Those with physical body ailments like acne or menstrual cramps, PMS or juvenile arthritis, IBS or headaches show up at my door. Also at the clinic are adolescents with cognitive challenges, ADD/ADHD and behavior problems. Some in this age group struggle with anxiety and/or depression, eating disorders or issues around self-esteem. Many are excessively stressed.

For some of these patients, it is a natural evolution from a challenging childhood filled with a history of many doctors, therapies and treatments; for others, the added stress of hormones and heightened expectations both at school and at home, seems to push the system in such a way, that symptoms begin to arise. There is not a significant difference in what I offer to this population, but there are ways of interacting, ways of communicating and ways of being supportive that draw on experience and skill. One thing I love about my work is coming into contact with people of all ages. But it is with teenagers that I feel I do my most creative work, gaining trust, speaking a particular language and consciously creating a unique relationship that can help this patient to get through whatever might be troubling them at the time of our visit. I also know that our time and work together may well influence a career choice and the way such a patient might think about medicine and healing for many years to come. I do not take this challenge lightly.

Like any group, teens come in all shapes, sizes and constitutional types, with all manner of chief complaints. I will share some general thoughts about treating teens based on my experience in practice and then offer up some patient examples from my work. I recently brought one of my own teens to a college campus for an elongated stay. As I helped him set up his room, he didn't really need the help, but he humored me by giving me jobs to hang up clothing and bring things in from the car. I saw at once how fleeting childhood is and how elements of adulthood are present from an early age. One child shows early the tendency to be organized or confident, one has an artistic bent or athleticism, another is exquisitely sensitive to people and surroundings. The small seed-like children grow in these in between years and further embody their natural tendencies. It seems the parents' main purpose in these teenagers' lives is to support them in the only *real* job they have: to figure out who they are and how they may best share their uniqueness and gifts with the world. And as they figure that out, to encourage the young adult to steadfastly stay true to that course and to know how to create a path to that truth and stick to it through years of experience, work, disappointments, the stuff of life. This narrow strip of adolescence offers medical providers a rare chance at helping steer young people in positive directions while offering a supportive ear to the sometimes overwhelmed parents. We ought never waste the chance.

Unless I believe that a teen's behavior is truly dangerous to themselves or others, I keep all information shared in the interview private; this includes drug/alcohol use and sexuality. If I feel that it might help the teen to talk about these issues with parents or other adults, I may give that advice or ask permission to share certain information. If I believe that the patient is in imminent danger, however, then I will share this information. I tell parents and teens about my confidentiality policy *before* we begin treatment so that we are all clear from the start. If they cannot abide by this policy, I have turned patients away, much as I've hated to do so.

Just as I wrote about earlier, the importance of parenting support is paramount. Issues such as limit setting and then shifting, offering privileges tied to responsibility taking, being firm but showing flexibility and raising the expectations around communication are all essential roles of parents of teenagers. Parents worry about many things; indeed, the stakes are higher now-a-days with regard to some of the dire consequences that loom, should a teen choose to engage in certain behaviors. With fewer community supports in place for parents of teens, worries mount. Some parents are working more, some are newly single, the camaraderie once felt at preschool drop-off or spontaneous playground conversations is gone; parents may no longer know who their teen is spending time with. Parenting can become a delicate dance parents do with their teens, while feeling clueless and isolated. Hopefully, the doctor's office can be one place parents turn for support, recommendations, appropriate referrals and especially, encouragement.

Younger teens often still want to have their parents join them in the visit. Older teens who are close with parents or who need help retelling medical histories may also prefer this. I do tell them that I might like a little time alone with each of them; there may be something one party wants to say without the other's presence. If the teen seems interested, I often take a minute or two to explain a little about my work and how I am most interested in the details of their illness and how they experience it. Most will not have heard many of the types of questions I pose and at the first visit, unless they are very extroverted, their answers may be brief or even unhelpful. Perhaps by the second or third visit, they will be better able to articulate specifics and particulars, because by then they understand what kind of information I am interested in.

Here are some things I look for when I see teen patients in the waiting room and in my office, which inform my understanding of them:

Interaction with parents. Some teens are still very much attached to parents, sitting close by, chatting with them; they may seem insecure or still quite child-like. If I see this in a 13 year old, it doesn't mean as much as if I see it in a 17 year old. When I see an overly insecure older teen, a handful of homeopathic remedies come to mind like *Pulsatilla* and *Baryta carbonica*. I would not prescribe such a remedy strictly on observation alone, but it might lead me to ask further questions about independence and confidence during my intake, when we get to the sections about temperament.

Interaction with siblings. Some teens totally disengage from younger siblings, some become automatic caregivers, some use siblings as constant sources of conflict expression, some are reluctant babysitters. Sometimes the teen is the younger sibling and I can see them looking up to a brother or sister; or they may ignore each other completely.

Interaction with office staff. An older teenage male might be flirting with my receptionist or another patient in the office, another teen might be chatting up the UPS delivery person, while another might be letting the parent do all the interacting with other adults in the waiting room. Some older teens come in by themselves and handle intake forms, payment. Because I have the pleasure of working in a small office, where I bring my own patients back from the waiting room, I am privy to some of these instances of potential social interaction. Sometimes these interactions are worth a lot in my understanding of the patient at hand. All of these sorts of observations give me clues into homeopathic constitutional remedy types and help inform the part of my casetaking about people-to-people interactions.

What they're reading. This can give an awful lot of information. Did they bring their own reading material? Is it science fiction, non-fiction, biography, a romance novel, or something they're studying at school? Or did they choose a magazine from our piles, and which one? This can give me some insight into passions and interests, which can help with conversational flow especially during the earlier part of the history taking.

What they're wearing. Lots of big clues here! Are they dressed creatively, provocatively, messily, grungily? Or do they seem to be dressed as their parents want them to be? Are they conscientious about small things or carefree? Is it all black or see-through and strapless? How high are the shoes? Are they dressed appropriately for the weather? Those teens who attend to every detail call to mind homeopathic remedies like *Natrum muriaticum, Thuja, Nux vomica* and *Carsinosinum* among others. This would not be sufficient information upon which to base a prescription, of course, and each remedy type is conscientious for different reasons, but such observations help guide my thinking and can give me information that dialogue may not always provide. I often tell students that observations are only as good as the questions they lead you to ask and this is never more true than when assessing the attire of a teenage patient.

What they're listening to. With the advent of personal music devices, I may have a chance to see what sort of music my patient enjoys listening to—and at what volume. Do they sing along, thump their hands, dance in their seat, close their eyes, or constantly switch stations or songs?

What else they're doing. I also notice what else they might be doing in the office—drawing, raiding the lollipop container, sleeping, chewing gum, eating candy, arguing with their parents, self-grooming. If they are eating or drinking, I pay attention to what it is and whether they are doing so surreptitiously or with gusto, neatly or messily, sharing or in private. I recall one gal who was plucking her eyebrows in my waiting room. I found this very strange. She was brought in for chronic diarrhea. In the end, she responded well to the homeopathic remedy, *Sulphur*. Those who respond well to this particular remedy often, among many other things, do not really care what other people think about them. Not sure how the remedy effected that in her, and after all it really was not a symptom, but her chronic digestive and bowel problems were cured!

Noticing physical appearance, here are some other things related to the teen's physical appearance that I am aware of and which may inform my case taking questions:

Posture. Posture says a lot about physical strength, basic anatomy and self-esteem. Attitude can also be reflected in posture and gait.

Skin. I look at the skin—is it smooth and baby like? Is there acne? Is there facial hair? Are they shaving?

Hair. I check out the hair—something within many teens' control and often used as a form of self-expression and style. This includes the amount of hair (zero to a lot), the shape and style, the various colors and whether it is groomed at all. I had an older male teen patient with a shaved head and tattoos along his neck, much to his mother's horror. His problem was asthma; he did well with a dietary shift away from dairy and refined foods, and with a group of botanical medicines to nourish lung tissue and decrease inflammation and with the constitutional homeopathic remedy, *Medorrhinum*, and the tattoo remains!

Make-up. I look for make-up. What kind and how much? Is it applied skillfully or just slapped on? Does it match the rest of the appearance?

Piercings. I look for piercings, which have become more and more popular. It is not unusual now for me to see pierced noses, navels, eyebrows and tongues, as well as many holes on all parts of the ear in teens of any age. As an aside, I have had a number of patients with naval piercings who develop vague but constant abdominal pain that improves when the jewelry is removed. I have also had several patients with abnormal mammograms who had lesions suspected around the nipple. These women had had in their earlier years nipple piercings.

Tattoos. I have seen teens with tattoos on the breast, buttock, ankle, back, wrist, arm, neck, behind the ear and shoulder. Some do it to rebel, others to express themselves; some succumb to peer pressure while sober or under the influence.

I have a policy in the office: I never act shocked at anything and I always ask about what I see. When did you do that? Did it hurt? Why did you do it? Would you do it again? That way I can get a sense of whether the teen has regrets or whether that choice is still reflecting something important to them.

So for instance, if a teen is dressed in many layers of clothing during warm weather, I ask whether they are chilly, are covering up, or just like to be cozy. I don't take anything at face value and I am not judging. Every symptom, every outward manifestation of the person is context dependent; you have to understand the why just as much as you have to understand the face value. In fact, there is almost no face value without the context.

A teen's attitude can be expressed by a whole range of things, many of which have already been mentioned. It may reflect how they feel about being in the office that day (e.g.,what they had to miss in order to be there) or it may be a more general expression of their underlying attitudes about life.

Another big clue to their attitude has to do with how I feel about the patient. Some patients I feel sorry for, some I feel annoyed by, some I 'connect' with, some I don't. I do not prescribe based solely on my own feelings about the patient, but neither do I ignore them. I use any information I perceive via observation or by my kinesthetic experience to inform the questions I ask.

Everyone goes through a tremendous transition from childhood to teenager—for some it is more difficult than others. From a homeopathic point of view, some kids stay the same remedy type, going from a sweet *Pulsatilla* kid to a sweet *Pulsatilla* teenager, no doubt becoming a lovely *Pulsatilla* adult. Others experience the adolescent years as if a huge volcano is erupting inside and this manifests on many levels; they go through various remedy types within a few years. Some of these patients seem unrecognizable to their parents, friends, relatives and homeopath!

I remember the first time I had this experience. I had treated a young girl for chronic earaches when she was seven to eight years old, and she had done very well on *Calcarea carbonica*, then *Sulphur* over the course of two years. I had not seen her for some time, when at the age of 14 she was brought in by her concerned mother for suicidal depression. When I went out to greet her (and mind you, she had been a ruddy, open-faced girl with a sunny disposition), I was met by a girl dressed entirely in black, including black nail polish, black eyeliner, and black lipstick. She was wearing a black t-shirt, ripped into shreds until just below the breast, and her hip-hugger pants were millimeters above her pubic hair. Her hair was greasy and completely covering her face, that is, the part that wasn't teased up into a sort of dread-locked beehive. She wore six inch black platform boots and towered over me as she walked (skulked) into my office.

I was overwhelmed. Where had that sweet little girl gone? Where was all that openness and love of life? I had to regroup quickly. Thankfully, she was tremendously helped with the remedy *Medorrhinum* and then *Aurum metallicum* and is now a graceful, worldly, college alumna.

Most teens that I have treated with these kinds of problems have come from families where there has been tremendous family stress such as divorce, death of a parent, extramarital affairs in the parents, a move to a new home during key years of friendships and courting, or serious financial problems. Of course, a history of depression or drug and alcohol abuse in the parents can also be a contributing factor. Even though parents may have been sober for many years, their children are more at risk for the same behaviors, much to parents' deep regret. Occasionally I see a teen like this in which none of the above family problems seem to be an issue. This always leads me to the statement: we do our best as parents and sad to say, there are no guarantees.

That teenagers are expressing anger, rage, inappropriate behaviors, and downright acts of violence is not new. I truly believe, however, that the media is not helping in these situations, but rather tends to create a culture that is numb to acts of violence and to the impact of such movies, television shows, music and advertisements—of which most Americans consume a steady diet.

For me, the most difficult patients are the ones who seem shut off from everything; I have to find some way *in* for these kids, especially if they really don't want to be there and are getting into trouble at home and at school. I try to loosen things up by talking about anything I know they may have some interest in or had some interest in (tipped off by parents). I try to name what I'm feeling because they're probably feeling it too, for example, 'It's really a bummer to have to be here, isn't it?' or 'Let's try to do this quickly so you can get back to whatever it is you'd rather be doing.'

I have also had the immeasurable pleasure of treating teens who, though they may have certain physical ailments or psychological issues, have tremendous creativity and energy, compassion and vision, who give me every hope that the world is moving in the right direction. With successful treatment, I am heartened to see passions ignited, social skills honed, and improved ability to synthesize information and experiences toward positive ends. I take a kind of vicarious pride in their strong curiosity about the world and their brave experiences and accomplishments, large and small.

It is not different treating teenagers, although it sometimes requires a bit more sleuthing and the willingness to see the patient as a full person with their own interests, passions, personalities, and quirks—maybe not quite what the parent had in mind. I need to put the things observed in proper context and perspective with the rest of the case, and prescribe from there. I try very much to enjoy these patients; they are the future adults of my practice and our world!

College Bound

When I had three older teens under one roof, I began to create a natural medicine packing list for when my kids would take that big step out the front door and into apartment/dormitory living or for when they struck out for some adventuresome travel. A few years back, I hand-wrote and hand-bound three copies of a small book called *Mom's Home Remedies*—one for each child. I may publish this little ditty one day. As it has turned out, being armed to help oneself when away from home comes in handy and an unforeseen eventuality is that other young people in need now seek out my children for advice. They are *not* dispensing medicines from their school lockers or dormitory rooms—but it makes me glad to hear that they are at least thinking about natural medicine solutions for what ails the people in their lives. They may never have wanted to go the doctoring route of their two parents, but lo and behold, it has come to them.

After raising my children with wholesome diets and when needed, natural therapies, it would be odd to imagine them reaching for conventional medicines for the first-aid and acute health problems that are bound to arise once living on their own. Increasingly, they as well as the teens and parents of teens in my practice ask me for natural medicine help in order to offer assistance to buddies for everything from menstrual cramps to headaches, allergies to poison ivy. If you, too, are getting ready to pack your teenager off to college or on their first trip away from home, what natural medicines should you send along?

Essential Natural Medicines

Acidophilus: This and other probiotics help keep the normal bacterial flora in balance in the digestive, gynecological and urinary tracts; it is also good for yeast infections in young women. I would send the kind of probiotic that doesn't need to be refrigerated.

Bromelain: Derived from pineapple, this enzyme is excellent for sports injuries like muscle strains and sprained ankles; it can also help to thin mucus and reduce inflammation during an acute upper respiratory illness.

Charcoal Tablets or Capsules: Charcoal can offer relief to the student suffering from dietary indiscretion, strong gas, bloating or food poisoning. For the student with a sore throat, sucking on charcoal tablets (not capsules) can help to pull infection away. Make sure your child is aware that ingesting activated charcoal will cause the stool to turn black temporarily and that it's not a cause for concern. Charcoal is not appropriate for long-term ingestion and can interfere with the absorption of certain pharmaceuticals including the birth control pill. Be sure your young adult knows this.

Vitamin C and Zinc: I tell my children to take Vitamin C and Zinc when starting to feel under the weather or when living in close proximity to others who are ill. This vitamin and mineral help to boost immune system function and helps the person fight off impending infection.

Vitamin-Mineral-Botanical Complex: There are many such general vitamin-mineral-botanical medicine complexes available that are excellent for helping bolster immune function. I like one called Vita-biotic (made by Eclectic Institute, Gresham, Oregon) which contains Magnesium, Zinc, Bioflavonoids, Echinacea, Garlic, Myrrh, Ginger, Cayenne, and Vitamins A, C, and B-6. I would instruct the person in need to take it as directed to prevent illness after exposure to others who are sick or at the first signs of feeling run down. It can also be used therapeutically for a cold, sinusitis, bronchitis, or earache. Such complexes help the body do its work of fighting illness-causing bacteria or viruses.

Most of the these natural medicine products listed here are available at natural food stores, so depending on where your young person lands, they can likely find these supplements when needed. With the widespread use of cell phones and email, directions can easily be delivered should problems arise.

But a sick child away from home for the first time may not have the wheels or the wherewithal to find these products, so it's nice to be prepared. If unopened, most of these natural medicines can remain effective for months while retaining their potency. That's why I have created a traveling first-aid kit in a small storage box that can be easily placed under a bed or on the top shelf of a closet. I have the homeopathic remedies; a small reference book, the botanical medicines and vitamins all packed away in this box—so it's in one place and readily available should any need arise.

If you know your child's constitutional remedy (i.e., the one homeopathic remedy, typically prescribed by a professional, that has helped your child's main symptoms and overall level of health on a number of occasions), then I would make sure you send them off with a few doses of that remedy in the 30c, 200c, and 1M potencies, just to have on hand. Should an illness arise, I would encourage my child to consult with the homeopath who initially prescribed that remedy to see if another dose of the remedy would be in order. Many times, a simple repetition of the constitutional remedy can give just the support the body needs to get over a particular injury or illness—especially if the person's physical general symptoms (body temperature, food cravings, thirst and basic temperament) have not shifted markedly during an illness *and* the symptoms of the acute illness are included in the indications for that constitutional remedy.

Being in a new situation, eating different food, and being exposed to a new set of germs are all *stressors* to the system, so it would not be unusual for a young person to succumb to illness in the first months of being away. That's why I try to see such patients *before* they take off—just to check in with them and perhaps give them a dose of their constitutional remedy.

A small first-aid homeopathic medicine kit with a simple, easy-to-follow list of indications would be a wonderful going-away present for any person leaving home. A variety of well-packaged kits are available for sale from homeopathic pharmacies, and since homeopathic remedies have a very long shelf life (they last indefinitely when stored under normal conditions), such a kit could become the basis of a student's future home pharmacy, years down the road.

With respect to potency/strength, I prefer the 30c potency for a first-aid kit because this potency is strong enough to help and to have lasting effects for most people with acute illnesses. I would also send along the first-aid book, *Homeopathic Medicine at Home* by M. Panos, MD, and J. Heimlich, which is easy to use and covers most of the basic acute health problems that arise.

If my son or daughter fell ill at school, I would encourage them to prescribe for their illness on as broad a basis as possible; that is, if I were supporting them by phone or email, I would try to glean information for a full homeopathic case, developing a complete profile of their symptoms on all levels—mental, emotional and physical. That said, oftentimes, keynote prescribing (where remedies are chosen based on just a few key symptoms of both the remedy and the patient) can be helpful for first-aid and acute situations.

Below, I have listed some of the remedies most commonly found in 30 remedy and 50 remedy kits on the market today, plus a few of the common indications for using these remedies. This will give you a sense of the sorts of ailments a person might try to help themselves with while living away from home.

Aconite for the first signs of any inflammation, the very beginning of a cold or sore throat; it can abort or shorten the duration of an illness.

Apis for swelling and redness from bug bites or poison ivy.

Arnica for trauma, inflammation and bruising, and for the stronger-than-usual sports injury.

Argentum nitricum for the student with stage fright or diarrhea from anxiety.

Arsenicum album for an attack of food poisoning; it may also be useful for many other acute inflammatory responses (for example colds and flu) where the student feels cold, wants warm drinks, has burning pain and feels anxious.

Belladonna for the first stages of inflammation where there is a feeling of heat and throbbing, usually accompanied by a fever, and where the person has glassy eyes and wide open pupils.

Bryonia alba for acute upper respiratory illnesses or musculoskeletal complaints, typically accompanied by aching, dryness throughout, constipation, irritability and heightened thirst.

Gelsemium for flus or colds that leave the sufferer wiped out, exhausted, with heavy eyelids, and perhaps a headache; also useful for anxiety before a test or performance.

Ignatia for the bad sore throat that is better from eating rough food; and of course, this remedy is also useful for the inevitable first heartbreak.

Kali bichromicum for sinusitis with thick discharges and headaches occurring in small spots over the eyes.

Lycopodium for digestive upset, gassiness and irritability.

Mercurius vivus for upper and lower respiratory tract complaints that are accompanied by excess salivation, lots of green-yellow mucus, and excessive perspiration.

Nux vomica for dietary indiscretion or overindulgence in alcohol (hangover); also for occasional constipation, irritability and upper respiratory infection with much runny nasal discharge.

Pulsatilla especially for the homesick son or daughter who cries easily and has a difficult time with separation from home (and may also have a cold with lots of bland yellow discharges).

If I knew that my child tended toward certain kinds of acute illnesses that respond to particular remedies, I would be sure that those remedies were contained in the kit. I would also include any other natural medicines that might be relevant for the young adult in need. For instance, if I had a daughter who was susceptible to urinary tract infections, I would be sure the kit contained the homeopathic remedies *Staphysagria, Causticum, Belladonna* and *Cantharis* as these remedies have an affinity for helping issues in that region. Each would be prescribed with particular specifications which I might also send along. I would also make sure she had an herbal tincture that contained botanical medicines good for the bladder, such as Slippery Elm and Cranberry.

If I knew my son or daughter was often injured in athletic pursuits, I would be sure the kit contained *Arnica, Rhus tox, Ruta* and *Bryonia*. I would also be sure to pack the herbs Bromelain and Curcumin, both excellent for reducing inflammation, preventing adhesion formation and helping to reduce lactic acid build up in the muscles.

Lastly, for the mothers, fathers and siblings left behind, it's good to recognize that this transition—no matter how carefully planned for, no matter how ready both child and parent are—is a stress. We homeopaths often notice that a patient's chronic symptoms flair up in the months surrounding a departure. We see stress as having potential impact on the physical, mental or emotional body and know that each of us tends to react to stress in patterned, almost predictable ways. Scheduling a routine visit around such times of transition, even if things seem to be going well, is always a good idea.

It is an odd job-description, that of parent. You pour your heart and soul into the raising of your children, dedicate endless hours, broad ranging resources and countless moments of worry—and then, poof! Fledge them from the nest. It is the right order and the appropriate next step at some point for most families in our culture, whether it is sending a young adult off to college, work, travel or just to live out from under the roof they have always known. But knowing that does not make the job any easier!

Still, packing your child off with a small box filled with a few tools and remedies to help them when illness might occur can give parents at least a tiny bit of comfort. And then, of course, when the last one(s) are off, the new phase of life begins for the parent, hopefully full of discovery and adventure, inside and out, time for reflection and the transferring of energy into one's own interests and passions.

Homeopathy from the Sidelines

In my years as the mother of three teenage athletes, fall season often found me sitting on the sidelines cheering, providing water and oranges to the players, offering free coaching advice to any spectators who would listen, and occasionally being asked to play team doctor. Our family enjoys these athletic events, which offer a good balance to academic pressures while allowing the players to keep in shape and experience the feeling of team camaraderie. In addition, we parent-fans have the opportunity to socialize and help out where we can. The first-aid kit in my car sees a fair amount of action come fall, though I more often offer an ice pack or a Bandaid than a homeopathic remedy.

Apart from actual sports injuries, most of the problems that arise have to do with over-exertion, dehydration, and too much sun and for some, over training. These can be bad combinations for serious athletes who may have neglected the need for extra water, sunscreen, nourishing food and keeping cool. Using beverages that help replenish electrolytes like Gatorade, or the somewhat more natural Recharge, is helpful. For a more in-depth chapter on sports, sports injury and sports psychology, see the chapter, 'I Want to be in the Olympics' on page 297.

Some of 'that stuff'

When a player is injured, it's not uncommon for a parent to come over and ask me for some of 'that stuff.' With the parent's request or permission, I give the homeopathic remedy *Arnica montana* when there has been any sort of hard blow, collision, sprained ankle or dislocated joint. People with these kinds of injuries will often need a different remedy over the course of the next few days, but it is reasonable to start them off with *Arnica.* So while we are applying ice and deciding whether a visit to the local emergency room is necessary, I will give the homeopathic remedy (I keep 30c potencies in my travel kit). I try to use these opportunities to educate parents about homeopathy and encourage them to bring their child in to my office some days or weeks later if they would like further help in supporting the healing process.

I have used *Glonoinum* to help an older teen who was nearing heatstroke—as evidenced by a ruddy face, vertigo and a throbbing headache. He recovered and was able to enjoy watching the rest of the game—although he was sidelined.

It's always good to have *Apis* on hand, as bees and wasps can find their way onto any athletic field. If the sting swells up quickly, looks red and feels better with ice, *Apis* would be your first choice. If that doesn't seem to help, try *Ledum*, which is helpful for puncture wounds, including those from insects.

I have offered *Magnesium phosphoricum* to players with severe leg cramps, along with advice on how to stretch the area and massage it, so that they can get past the cramps and back into the game.

Natural Remedies and Common Sense

I recall one sweet teenager who suddenly became very nauseated at a game, feeling like she would vomit, probably due to a combination of over-exertion, pressure to perform, and running hard and long. I didn't have my remedies nearby that day, but in my first-aid kit I did have candied Ginger, which she sucked on. She took a moment to collect herself and was back in action a short while later. It's easy to carry Ginger candy, and kids like the taste. But you can use Ginger in any form you happen to have (for example fresh, tablets, tea, soda, cookies) to help settle an upset stomach.

For those kids who develop blisters (especially during long tournaments) or who come to games with them, we apply moleskin to the area around the blister to reduce the pressure. I always bring extra socks, both the sort that wick moisture away from the skin and plain athletic socks. Sore, blistered feet can feel a lot better with dry socks.

Where there is inflammation and swelling, in addition to giving the homeopathic remedy indicated, I will advise parents to go to the health food store and purchase two natural anti-inflammatory supplements: Bromelain, an enzyme derived from pineapple, and Curcumin, derived from turmeric. I recommend 500 mg of each, two to three times a day, to be taken together between meals.

From the sidelines, I do not treat those with chronic conditions who are having exacerbations during a game. A child with asthma, allergies or chronic musculoskeletal problems, for example, is best seen in the office. They require a full homeopathic intake, assessment, and follow-up.

Sports First-aid Kit

My basic first-aid sports kit goes somewhat beyond a mini homeopathic pharmacy, so I'm ready for most minor problems that arise. It includes:

- Ice packs
- Bandaids, small and large
- Tweezers
- Antibiotic ointment
- Calendula salve
- Powdered Gatorade or other electrolyte replacement
- Ginger candy
- Protein bars
- Sunblock
- Extra socks
- Moleskin and small scissors
- Homeopathic remedies: *Arnica, Aconite, Apis,*

Arsenicum, Belladonna, Bryonia, Cantharis, Carbo vegetabilis, Glonoinum, Hypericum, Ledum, Magnesium phosphoricum, Rhus toxicodendron and Ruta graveolens

Generally speaking, injuries sustained during sporting events also need time to heal. Nevertheless, we sidelined parents and fans have much to offer the injured athlete. We can support their healing with natural medicines with good results and few side effects. So play hard, play fair, and have fun!

Chapter 5

For Adults

Back to School Stress for Mom(Poison Ivy Story)

Swede, a lovely blue-eyed woman, bright and effusive, had been a patient of mine for fifteen years. Although she had weathered her share of acute illness and some brushes with more serious pathology, she was enjoying good health as she entered her middle years and was bracing, with equal portions of trepidation and enthusiasm, for the transition to an empty nest. The youngest of her four children was about to be fledged, off to a far-away Ivy League college in the fall.

Swede called me one morning at the crack of dawn as I was puttering in the fall garden, gathering the last of the raspberries and inhaling the bittersweet end of summer as it marched across my yard. She apologized profusely for calling early, calling me at home, and calling me at all, but she had the worst case of poison ivy, and it was either call me, or go to the local emergency room. I had office appointments beginning a few hours later, so I asked if she could meet me there at lunchtime when I would have a few free minutes. Emboldened by her pain and anxiety, this usually mild mannered woman pushed: maybe she could come in before my first patient? How forward, I thought, but being immersed in the gentleness of morning dew, I acquiesced.

Like many practitioners, I have seen cases of poison ivy that truly take the breath away. I have observed large tracts of skin with excoriation, weeping and crusting. I have seen faces blown up, nearly unrecognizable and limbs distorted by swelling. I have been privy to genital exfoliation and plantar disintegration, all from the effects of this ubiquitous and pesky weed.

When Swede met me later that morning, she presented none of the above. Instead, what I saw when she gingerly rolled back her gauzy cotton sleeve, was a small strand of pearly vesicles, no more than two inches long. There was an even smaller satellite lesion with perhaps three tapioca-like dots. I kept looking farther up the arm for the dramatic presentation I had been expecting, the effects of this demon at work ... but, there was nothing more!

With unadulterated urgency, Swede described her intense pain, her sleeplessness and the pure agony she was experiencing. It was, I am sorry to say, difficult to believe! Doctors are trained never to make faces, never to let our expressions betray our thoughts. But my mouth was surely hanging open. I felt a bit confused and said, "I don't know ... it just really doesn't look that bad."

Swede said she knew it didn't look bad, but it really was horrible and she couldn't stand it another minute. She had self-prescribed the homeopathic remedy *Rhus toxicodendron* 12c that morning and reported that she did feel somewhat better. So I sent her home with some of the same medicine in higher doses, and with instructions to call me later in the day, at the office.

Between patients, reviewing charts, I received Swede's teary call. It was much worse, she was much worse. Incapable of sitting still and unable to get a grip on herself, she was scurrying around the house, feeling hot and breathless. I asked her to do me a favor: try a cold compress to the area and let me know how it felt. She reported that it gave a little temporary relief. I then asked her to do the same with a hot one. As she laid that hot cloth on the eruptions, she let out a screeching yelp, as if she had placed her whole arm on top of a sizzling hot, wood-burning stove. She began to cry in earnest—wracking sobs, which I listened to as empathetically as telephone technology allows.

I asked a few more questions. She described a searing pain, as if someone was torturing her, dragging a not-quite-extinguished match along the tender flank of her wrist. She said she had to keep moving, literally without rest. If she stopped, the excruciating pain was exacerbated.

I have seen people who need one particular homeopathic remedy arrive at such a point as the state that Swede was in—with arthritis, with burns, with insect bites, and yes, with poison ivy. I told Swede to take *Apis mellifica* 30c and call me in the morning.

When I went home that evening and spent time in the yard with my children, I was cautioning them, "Don't go in there, there's poison ivy ... Leave that ball, we'll get another one. ... Don't touch that vine!" Call me paranoid.

Swede did call the next day, bright and early, to say she

was all better. No pain. Nada. I asked if the eruption was gone and she said it was still there, but it no longer hurt. She was planning to go to work that day, and oh yes, thanks!

Incredible that a little pellet of medicine can work so deeply, so quickly, that someone writhing in pain can be fine a few hours later, just like that! We think about using the remedy *Apis mellifica* when the problem at hand has the modalities of being both better from cold and worse from heat. There is typically swelling of the part in question. People who need *Apis mellifica* are usually restless and irritable, and they seem quite sensitive to their pain or discomfort. Their problems are often worse at night.

In addition, when *Apis mellifica* is indicated, I find that it is not uncommon to see some sort of shift in the home life, and the attendant anxiety that accompanies it as a precursor to the *Apis mellifica* state. You see, there was tremendous stress at home for Swede. As she was helping her youngest pack and get ready to take a giant step away from home, what should have been a small acute illness took on grandiose proportions. This was the way mother Swede apparently somatosized her sad and mixed emotions, and was then able to jump into empty-nesthood without the tremendous emotional upheaval that sometimes accompanies such transitions. Though the poison ivy caused an unpleasant few days, in a sense, you might say that Swede took much of her angst and worry and compressed it into this pathology.

It is lovely to treat a first-aid or acute problem with homeopathy as part of a practice in which I largely see those with chronic disease. The very sick get well, too, but seldom as dramatically and completely as those with acute problems like Swede.

So bring on those acutes! In times of back-to-school changes for children and those who care for them, we often see the stress of such transitions manifesting in physical ailments. I am reminded to think of those kinds of stressors as part of the possible etiology or cause, when treating people at such times in their lives.

The Perfect Mother

The two children that Kitty brought to see me were adorable. A four year old girl with chronic earaches and allergies and an eight year old daughter with anxiety and skin problems were dressed impeccably and wore matching handmade capes. I was struck by how obedient the children were, sitting quietly during exams and listening well to mother. Over the course of a year I worked with the girls to get them back on track. As I had the opportunity, I could see that the mother was struggling with the enormous load of motherhood. She was at home with the children, committed to feeding the family an organic foods diet, to home-schooling and to keeping a tidy home. The wear on her showed in her anxiety and worry, in her clear fatigue and in what I thought looked like feelings of overwhelm. When I suggested that maybe it was time for her to make an appointment, she broke down crying. I think she felt at once like I could tell she was losing her grasp but also happy that someone expressed concern.

At 38, this former laboratory technician had known a full, busy and satisfying life before children. She never imagined herself as an at-home mother, but after the birth of her daughter she became disconcerted at the idea of someone else caring for her perfect daughter. She nursed on demand and enjoyed a family bed. By the time she became pregnant again three years later, she knew she was in for the long haul and would do everything in her power to raise, feed, care for and educate her own children. Her efforts had been noble but alas, she was decompensating, an unfortunate victim of her own high standards.

Increasingly I see families where this is the case. The lofty ideals of raising a family without television, without prepared food, without outside help leaves the mothers, and sometimes the stay-at-home father overwhelmed, exhausted and disappointed in themselves. Of course the job of being home raising a family was never meant to be done in isolation or without the support of family, friends and community nearby. But our society has pockets where based on religious beliefs, geography or personal temperament, some individuals who start out this way, find ultimately that it is not sustainable.

For Kitty, her own tendencies towards obsessive compulsive disorder came into play and were heightened after the birth of her children. She was unable to let go of the cleaning routine, and was unable to lower her standards about orderliness and excellence. She could spend hours after the children were in bed, cleaning and organizing. She judged herself harshly if she felt she was not doing everything and doing it well. Her husband was supportive and helped out where he could, but he worked long hours to support their decision that Kitty would be home with the children.

Theoretically Kitty wanted to involve her children with all kinds of enrichment opportunities and the ability to meet and spend time with other home-schooling families, but alas, Kitty herself found filling the weekly schedule with activities and classes and social engagements to be too overwhelming. Never one to be comfortable in social settings, these group efforts were exhausting and anxiety producing for her. As she put it, her lack of confidence and general insecurity made just being with others stressful. She would rather be home with her two children, learning together, baking, sewing, doing art projects or playing in the yard. In some ways this approach worked for Kitty as she could control all aspects of the environment for herself as well as for her children.

The only problem is that it became exhausting. Kitty had a life-long issue with fatigue, needing daily afternoon naps of 1-2 hours. She would wake in the mid-afternoon refreshed but would soon be tired again. In any case, doing everything to run a household, educate and entertain children was wearing her thin.

Kitty also described a life long relationship with depression though as she sat before me, she seemed eager, almost anxious, with eyes wide open and an easy ability to connect with me one-to-one. She reported she was not a laid back person, rather often anxious. Social settings were the worst where she would replay interactions and wonder constantly if she had said or done the right things. She was severely averse to discord and could not bear the idea of someone being upset with her. At home, she felt her OCD-like behaviors the most. She might check or recheck things in the house such as light switches and the toaster, to make sure they were off or unplugged. She had very little in the way of a support system with family far away both geographically and emotionally.

Since adolescence, Kitty struggled with severe cystic acne; in the past few years her skin was 'falling apart,' with outbreaks all across her forehead, nose area and chin as well as her back and chest. The blemishes were red, raised and coalesced into large patches. There was an angry look to the skin that Kitty, though not especially vain, was aware of, especially as children would often ask her what was wrong with her face. She did not try to cover up the areas, and had tried any number of over the counter treatments to no avail. The only treatment that had ever had an impact was antibiotic therapy, but Kitty could not tolerate it on her digestive system, so she had discontinued treatment after several months, many years before.

Kitty tended to be constipated and controlled the issue with diet and keeping well hydrated. Her review of systems was otherwise unremarkable.

When I looked at Kitty, I had the benefit of having known her for over a year and of watching her as a mother with her children when she brought them in for their visits. She was always attentive, loving and firm with her kids and they all seemed to love each other very much. The younger daughter had done very well with the remedy *Silicea*, which addressed both her earaches and allergies and her sister had done well with the remedy *Sulphur*. Sometimes we do see remedies running through families, but of course, the case must be taken in full and analyzed as its own story.

Kitty's shy and insecure temperament, her OCD-like behaviors and social anxiety coupled with the nature of her physical complaints, led me to the remedy *Silicea*. That her daughter had done very well on that remedy was a good confirmatory thing for me, but I would have given Kitty *Silicea* regardless. When I repertorized Kitty's case, the other remedies that came through strongly and that I seriously considered were: *Arsenicum album, Carsinosinum,* and *Causticum*. She had the anxieties and physical general symptoms of *Arsenicum album*, the remedy I felt came closest to matching her symptoms, but in the end I felt the root of her issues was her weakness which drove her to create many structures and rules to compensate for her fatigue and overwhelm as opposed to trying to control her environment out of fear and anxiety, which would point more to *Arsenicum album*.

I gave Kitty *Silicea* 200c and also a number of things to help with the acne. Because she had had a positive response locally, i.e., on her skin, from antibiotics in the past, I decided to give her a natural anti-bacterial in the botanical medicine/vitamin supplement form. I gave her a product called Optibiotic made by Eclectic Institute which contains vitamin A, C, B-6, magnesium, Zinc, Bioflavonoids, Echinaceae, Myrhh, Ginger, and capsicum. This is also sold in health food stores under the name VitaBiotic. I have had success with this combination supplement for a number of complaints including cystic acne. I also recommended she take a probiotic. We ordered blood work to rule out anemia and thyroid disease, due to her ongoing and extreme fatigue, but all tests came back in the normal range.

When Kitty came back, the first thing I noticed when she was sitting in the waiting room was her clear skin. She was thrilled too, for the first time in memory, have a clear complexion. There were still outbreaks on the chest and back, but her face was quite lovely. Kitty reported feeling more energy and more mental clarity. She hadn't realized what a fog she had been in, but felt somehow more energized and more motivated. She had taken on a home-school group event and was feeling good about being involved with that discrete event and several other mothers she would be interacting with in order to help organize, promote and run the afternoon experience.

At that point I did not repeat the remedy, but did have her stay on the other supplements. When I saw Kitty three months after the *Silicea*, she spoke about how she was feeling more comfortable in social settings, relaying a story about a holiday party from her husband's work which she generally would dread and how instead this year, she had made herself a new skirt for the occasion and had actually looked forward to attending and indeed enjoyed herself. She had for the first time since her children were born, hired a babysitter so she and her husband could go out. In short, she seemed to be loosening the reins a bit at home and better able to enjoy herself, her husband and her children.

I have continued to see Kitty over the ensuing years. Every so often she comes in feeling a bit low or a bit blue and I give her a dose of *Silicea 1M*, which seems to shore her up, put a little pep back in walk and allow her to relax a bit. We know that those who need *Silicea* tend to be a bit weak and therefore develop elements of rigidity to balance out that weakness. When we give the remedy, the weakness is ameliorated and so the rigidity – as in Kitty's case, all the rules, the OCD tendencies, etc., — too are lessened. After six months Kitty discontinued her supplements and her skin, including her back and chest, have remained clear.

Kitty is still doing all she was doing, but from a place of energy and conviction. Her daughter, now a teenager is thinking about attending the local high school and Kitty is entertaining all options, not feeling as inflexible about home-schooling her kids all the way through. In all, there is, as is appropriate as children get older, more give and take.

Sometimes when treating children, we can see that a parent would greatly benefit from a remedy or from advice and support. And sometimes it takes a year or two to build the confidence and trust needed to make such a suggestion. Treating families is almost always the best way to go, the insights you glean during case taking for one member influence our understanding of other family members' own stories. It is one of the most rewarding aspects of practice, seeing members across family lines, seeing how they relate and don't, seeing how they connect and don't and always keeping in the forefront of my analytic mind how those relationships impact and reflect particular constitutional types.

The *A Cappella* Singer Who Lost Her Voice

The first time I see Sally, her beautiful, red, wavy hair pulled away from her face with a barrette, but escaping here and there strikes me. It frames her features and gives her a peaceful and angelic look. Sally is up on her feet in no time when I greet her in the waiting room. I extend my hand, which she shakes with great vigor, an easy and warm smile on her face. She leads the way to my small private office, her hair waving along as she moves, with rhythm and shimmer. I can tell this will be a pleasurable first visit. It almost does not matter what her medical complaint is, I can tell she is an upbeat and high spirited person, which will make even a doctor visit enjoyable.

Sally is referred to me by a friend of a friend whose daughter was significantly helped by my recommendations for the treatment of long standing allergies. It is not greatly out of Sally's worldview to try something like naturopathic medicine. She is an outgoing, educated person with a natural curiosity about the world and openness to new things. She was dissatisfied with the care and attention she received over the past years for her problems and had not seen measureable results from those approaches. She felt she had nothing to lose.

When I look down at her chart, I read that her chief complaint is chronic laryngitis. For years, this 39 year old mother is unable to get through the winter months without becoming ill and losing her voice. She works as a music and movement teacher for little children and I imagine is very good at it. She adores the work, for the creative outlet it provides, the social interactions with young families and for the fact that she is planting musical seeds into the hearts and minds of a whole new generation. She sees how these young people absorb, at some level, even more than the high school chorus members she previously taught. Her career allows for a more flexible schedule, which enables Sally to spend more time with her own child. That said, when ill and constantly hoarse or even mute, she is left unable to sing and cannot easily modulate her voice to the task or group at hand; for several weeks at various intervals through the last number of winters, her work has become nearly impossible.

Having grown up in small town Vermont, the daughter of a factory worker and a secretary, she performed in many musical productions and sang in choruses throughout her childhood. While attending university, she joined an *a cappella* group, an activity and passion she retains these many years later. She was a founding member of an area all women's *a cappella* group so relies on her strong and resonant voice for both her livelihood as well as one of her life's greatest pleasures.

With rural Vermont roots (Sally told me that her home town population was less than the number of people in her first college dormitory), Sally is not unaccustomed to cold weather, but it seems that in recent years, the stress of the cold and perhaps the exposure to more germs from being around small children have left her susceptible and unable to effectively prevent or even treat these recurrent illnesses.

Over the previous two months she has been sick without relief. She develops a sore throat with swollen glands under her chin and then begins to lose her voice. She has an earache and a sensation of swelling in and around her ears. She has treated with antibiotics and decongestants to no avail. When tactics were switched to treating as if she suffered from an allergy, the medications recommended made her loopy and exhausted and more importantly, also did not help. She found losing her voice seriously unacceptable and when her voice returned, it retained a tinny and gravely element which was not something she could employ in any of her singing ventures. The postnasal drip and painful sinusitis were seriously disrupting her ability not only to earn a living, but to communicate at all.

Given all of that, I was surprised at how cheerful and upbeat Sally was. Her positive attitude impressed me and gave me confidence in her willingness to collaborate in whatever medical plan I would create for her. Temperament and attitude, two seemingly in-born characteristics are integrally connected with how the doctor/patient relationship will evolve. I aim to work hard for all my patients, some just make it a bit easier.

Sally told me that when her family doctor suggested yet another round of antibiotics, she suspected that approach was just not going to work. Encouraged by her friend, she made an appointment with me. She'd come to think that something was out of kilter with her ability to stem her ongoing infections, and perhaps an approach that took that into consideration would be more effective. She also wondered if perhaps she needed to find someone who could help her look at her overall health, someone who might see her throat/sinus/voice issues in context of her overarching health. She had come to the right place.

After taking Sally's complete patient history, I do a relevant physical exam and come to certain conclusions. It seems true that Sally is run down. It seems true that the antibiotics themselves may be making her more susceptible to getting sick, as they likely wipe out the good flora in the system which help us stay healthy. I made the following recommendations.

I asked Sally to take vitamin C, vitamin E and Zinc in doses appropriate to her weight, her condition and her diet and at times during the day related to her eating habits. I instructed her to check her multiple vitamin and be sure she would be receiving a minimal dosage of copper to help balance the extra Zinc. If it was not in that supplement, it would be added to her regimen; beta-carotene which is the vegetable source of vitamin A, was also recommended.

Each of these vitamins and minerals act to support the production and maintenance of healthy mucus membrane in the upper respiratory tract and each also helps to support a strong immune system function. I asked Sally to pick up some Slippery Elm lozenges, sold for the treatment of sore throat and which work well to directly sooth the irritated tissues in the area.

Finally, I suggested a combination vitamin/herbal supplement that I have used for 25 years with patients to help fight infection. I gave directions on how to take it should early warning symptoms of her laryngitis crop up. I also recommended the taking of a probiotic, to help replenish the normal flora in her digestive tract, which was likely wiped out by the recent overuse of antibiotics.

We discussed some dietary considerations, ways that Sally might side-step refined carbohydrates and simple sugars and what she might replace those with. I underscored the need for her to get plenty of rest and drink extra water during this time.

Lastly, I prescribed a constitutional homeopathic remedy, *Natrum muriaticum*. Homeopathy is a system of natural medicine designed to help bring balance and vitality and lessen presenting symptoms. I choose the remedy based on the way Sally experiences her problems, as well as how the chief complaint fits into her overall health. When deciding on a remedy, I also take in to account some of the general physical symptoms Sally has such as her overall body temperature, food cravings, sleep patterns and temperament. Homeopathic remedies are prescribed for a specific person, not for a particular diagnosis. I invited her to call me before our eight week follow up appointment if she had any questions or if any concerns arise.

I did not hear from her until I went to find her in the waiting room some two months later at our scheduled follow-up appointment. Sally told me that she had begun to feel better right away. Her voice had begun to sound more like her own and she no longer felt the bothersome post-nasal drip. She reported better energy. In short, Sally felt great. With a story like this, most would be very enthusiastic, but I was guarded in my excitement because we were in the warm summer months. Her exposure to small children was limited and she had more opportunities to be outside in the fresh air while doing things she enjoyed. Perhaps it was just coincidence. I would really only be satisfied with our work together if we could get Sally through a long New England winter with fewer infections or ones she could get through without antibiotics.

Indeed, I do not hear from Sally until some ten months later, when she comes in with a new problem. First, she wants me to know that the winter came and went with nary a laryngitis.

At the first sign of any discomfort, she reverted back to my previous recommendations and was able to nip in the bud any looming infection. She was thrilled. Her sleep and energy have never been better.

What brings her in is as an issue with gastric reflux. She's bothered by constant acid reflux regardless of what she eats or drinks. This new symptom is most unpleasant. I ask her to repeat the constitutional remedy, *Natrum muriaticum,* and give her a recommendation for deglycerinated glycerhizza (DGL), a preparation made from the licorice plant which helps to sooth and nourish the lining of the lower esophagus and stomach. She will take the DGL with meals and before bed. I also advise her to pick up with the Zinc and copper supplementation, which helps to build healthy mucus membrane in the area. Two days later her reflux symptoms were gone.

A year and a half after our first meeting Sally shares with me a funny fact. She says that I spent more time with her during our first interview than she has spent with her primary care doctor—in total, if you add up all of her visits to him over the course of her life. She marvels at the number and type of questions I asked. She mentions that she's told her husband how I was interested not just in her laryngitis but rather about *her*, how her illness is brought about, how she experiences it and how it impacts her family and life. She feels that I hear and understand her. That the recommendations were also successful is heartening to me, but that her personal experience in my office was pleasant, and reflected authentic and relevant communication, I am equally pleased to hear. Sally refers me many patients who have all manner of complaints. Though some of her friends think it strange that she sought care from a naturopathic doctor, she feels that her year and a half of not getting sick—the utter disappearance of laryngitis from her winters—speaks for itself. She plans to bring her son in for the prevention of chronic throat infections and I look forward to welcoming another member of her family into my practice. She would likewise encourage her husband to make an appointment for a nagging skin problem, but she says, "He is not quite ready to make the leap."

I practice in a state where I am licensed as a primary care physician and where many of my patients receive insurance reimbursement for my services. Yet comments like Sally's about her reticent husband even after my decades of practice, remind me that for some, natural medicine approaches still lie outside the mainstream medical model which in turn causes discomfort and resistance. Though many of my patients sought me out *because of* my training and expertise, others do not. The reluctance may stem from lack of knowledge and understanding about my education and scope of practice or from a bias against trying something new. I have treated large and extended families who only after ten or fifteen people in the family have benefited from my care, or after twelve or thirteen years, will the reluctant family elder show up, and sometimes then kicking and screaming. But we take all comers and hopefully even for the less than friendly, we can find an approach that works to improve health and vitality.

Sneezing and Yelling: Two Parts of the Whole Help with a Severe Case of Hay Fever

There are many times when a patient's chief complaint is clear and straightforward. It is easy for the patient to describe such strong and distinct symptoms, which in turn makes it easy for the homeopath to find the symptoms in the repertory, study the case and prescribe a remedy. Yet sometimes the remedy chosen by the homeopath does not work. In such cases, it is important to consider that a symptom may be representing a larger concept for that patient. When that larger concept is understood by the homeopath, it can be easier to understand the patient's case and to prescribe effectively.

When I take a case and have elicited a symptom, I ask myself, what is that symptom an example of? Are there other examples of that in the person's story? This helps both to inform my case taking and organize the information I get from the patient.

The case below illustrates how seeing the same underlying issue manifested on different systems of a patient will reinforce my understanding of him and improve my ability to prescribe correctly for him.

A 30 year old man came to see me, referred by his wife. He came reluctantly, not believing homeopathy could help the serious seasonal allergies that troubled him about half of each year.

He was well dressed, neat and punctual, and appeared to be a straight-talking, earnest young man. He seemed nervous during the interview, perhaps part of an overall anxiety or maybe more the sort of nervousness some people experience when meeting someone for the first time.

I took my time telling him how I enjoyed working with his lovely wife and three wonderful children, and how they seemed to be raising terrific kids. I explained a bit about my approach to medicine and answered his general questions. I always take time early in the interview to establish rapport with the patient and to set a welcoming and comfortable atmosphere in the consultation room.

The hay fever, which bothered him for several months both spring and fall, consisted of tremendous itchiness of the eyes, a runny nose and frequent bouts of explosive sneezing. The sneezing would come on all of a sudden, was intense and uncontrollable, and left him feeling extremely exhausted. The unpredictability and severity of his hay fever made it difficult for him to drive, to concentrate at work, or to plan outings. He had used all manner of over-the-counter medication with little to no success.

I wondered whether I might find other examples of explosiveness, so I began by asking general questions about his work and family life. He worked in the computer industry and enjoyed the responsibility and respect he earned on the job. He loved his wife and family, but found he had little patience for home life. He was irritable most of the time, easily angered by small things, and would find himself yelling at someone about something almost every day. Being a 'neat freak,' as he put it, did not help matters. He knew he was focusing on the wrong things, but he couldn't help himself. The mean, angry words would escape from his mouth before he had time to think. He would scream and sometimes throw things, frightening the children with his explosiveness. Afterwards he would feel exhausted and wiped out. The way in which he described his anger and irritability was very similar to how he had described his sneezing fits. The similar symptoms occurred, one in their physical realm and one more in the emotional sphere.

We often see symptoms in the physical and emotional spheres that mirror one another, as the Vital Force manifests imbalance in similar ways throughout the system. In this case, both the sneezing and the angry outbursts were examples of explosiveness. I organize my patients' symptoms accordingly; seeing how symptoms on various systems are similar helps me to receive the case without being overwhelmed by what might otherwise be understood as separate and distinct problems.

This patient kept a very strict routine and felt better if he was in control of his own time. To illustrate this point, he reported he'd rather be an hour early than a minute late—which of course, with a family of five, was a near impossibility. His wife was much more laid-back about most things, which he knew was good in terms of balance and running the household, but at the same time, it drove him crazy.

He tended towards constipation with two to three bowel movements per week, though he did have the urge to move his bowels most days. He desired spicy foods like chicken wings and salsa as well as beer and sweets. He drank some alcohol most days, a beer or two after work, and considerably more on the weekends. He did not see this as a problem, but according to his wife, it was an issue. It took him away from the family and made him inaccessible to her. He would retreat to the basement where he would work alone on his hobbies for long hours. To relax, he enjoyed re-organizing his tools or cleaning his workspace.

His sleep was frequently disturbed in the middle of the night with worries about work, finances, and remorse over his outbursts during the day. He was often chilly but perspired profusely, especially when feeling uptight.

When thinking about this man, his hay fever, and the way that fit into his overall health, emotionally and physically, I wanted to give a remedy that covered the whole case. Though the hay fever was troubling, we needed a remedy that would also address his issues of irritability, bad temper, self-control and remorse. One could prescribe a specific hay fever remedy such as *Sabadilla* or *Wyethia,* but when the whole person cries out for a remedy and that remedy also covers the physical symptomatology, it is always preferable to give the remedy that covers the whole case.

Looking at his overarching concerns (intense hay fever, irritability and anger, constipation, and insomnia) we recognize many of the key features of the remedy *Nux vomica.* Furthermore, his attention to detail, yearning for order, and need for control fit well into our understanding of this remedy. His strong and unpredictable temper, his excessive use of alcohol, and his tendency to be chilly further confirmed the prescription.

I prescribed *Nux vomica* 6c for him to take twice a day for one month. He was a heavy coffee drinker and I was concerned that he might antidote the remedy with all the coffee, yet it was clear he was not quite ready to stop the coffee, hence the low potency, with frequent repetition.

I saw him six months later, not my usual interval for a first follow-up, but some of my patients will only return when they are not doing well. He reported that he'd had no hay fever the previous season, and he could not remember the last time he'd had an angry outburst at home. He was quite pleased, if somewhat incredulous, about the effects of the homeopathic remedy. He had come in because he was beginning to feel a tickle in his throat and wanted to prevent the hay fever from returning. I repeated *Nux vomica,* this time in 200c potency, one dose, as he had stopped drinking coffee at some point in the last six months.

One year later, he returned to see me asking if he could have another dose of 'that stuff.' He'd been well physically, but was feeling the irritability creeping back. In addition to stopping coffee, he had cut way back on his alcohol consumption over the past year.

I hear of this patient intermittently from his wife, who was likewise pleased with the results. His ability to relax and be more present naturally impacted his whole family. Giving a remedy to help the hay fever, which is what had brought the patient into the clinic, clearly had a more widespread and most welcome influence.

This family has sent me many a hay fever sufferer over the years, some of whom fare as well, others of whom experience slower progress. In my experience, when we can see the hay fever, allergies, eczema or asthma as part of the whole person, when we understand the symptoms as examples of larger concepts and prescribe accordingly, we can almost always expect better results.

'Tis the Season to Be Stressed Out, Fa-la-la-la-la: A Case of Chronic Sinusitis

Every holiday season, the stresses of family gatherings, long distance travel and dietary indiscretions—coupled with high expectations and often let-down—take their toll on the health of many celebrators. Weeks of anticipation, extra food preparation, house cleaning and gift making or buying leave many people exhausted and burned out, even before the holidays begin.

At this time of year, I try to impress on my patients that, just as in homeopathy, less is more. I encourage my vulnerable patients, especially those who always seem to get sick right in time for the big days, to lower their expectations, choose a few traditions that are dear to them, and stop trying to do everything for everyone. We review the health-building things they can do, at home and on the road, to ensure that they are as strong as possible going into this season. We try to figure out how they can keep exercise as well as things that help them relax on the top of their 'to-do' lists, even when they feel pressed for time. Ultimately, it is my hope that they will be able to experience the joys and connections of the season in good health.

Loren, a mother of three under the age of five, came to see me almost ten years ago when she was thirty-two. Her main issue was chronic sinusitis with a low grade but bothersome sense of fullness in her frontal and maxillary sinuses as well as chronic post-nasal drip. She experienced this feeling of fullness year-round, but at times, it would progress to incapacitating sinus headaches. In addition, Loren suffered from intermittent bouts of acute, severe sinusitis. For the chronic condition, she had taken years of allergy medications and allergy shots. For the acute infections, she had often received antibiotics, which would address the severe situation but would leave her feeling unwell and completely exhausted.

Using appropriate constitutional homeopathic care along with some gentle naturopathic therapies, Loren has done fairly well over the last ten years. During the first year of treatment, her chronic sensation of sinus fullness and attendant headaches gradually went away. Her post-nasal drip also became a thing of the past, and she was thrilled with these results.

Every year come November, however, things would begin to fall apart for Loren. As soon as the weather changed and the windows in her house were closed, her sensitivities to cold, dust, mold, and dampness were triggered. On top of that, the stress of hosting Thanksgiving for her extended family and the enormity of Christmas heading her way would just about pull her under.

In these times of acute illness, Loren would develop tremendous pain over her cheekbones in her maxillary sinuses. She had copious, thick, clear discharge from her nose, which also caused post-nasal drip. As her head filled up, the headache would come on and she would have to find a dark, quiet room in which to lie down. That, of course, wasn't really possible with three small children to tend, so Loren would become irritable and short tempered, quite different from her usual calm and loving self. Whenever she got sick like this, she would also be plagued with canker sores on her lips and nose. She describes years of family holiday portraits in which she looked terrible—full of red, spreading lip sores.

Aside from her sinus troubles, Loren has enjoyed excellent health. Fastidious and organized, she concerns herself with the smallest details of her home, kitchen and children. We won a small victory when I convinced her that not ironing her children's t-shirts was really okay! (I recounted the story of my now grown daughter, who at age 7 was asked by an overnight guest where her mom kept the iron and responded, 'What's an iron?') I urged Loren to work with her husband to find a few extra dollars to afford some childcare, if even only a few hours a week, and to treat herself before the holidays by hiring someone to help share the cleaning. Because it is important to Loren that she hand-make holiday gifts for each of her siblings and their children, we brainstormed possible projects that would be heartfelt but not terribly time-consuming. Baking suited her and she found that it was a gift she could imbue with love and feel good about giving, without being overburdened by it.

For the first several years of our work together, I saw Loren every few months to check in, fine-tune some of the naturopathic protocols, and prescribe a homeopathic remedy if needed. More recently, she feels so much better that she rarely needs to see me. But each year around October, we do have a standing date. She comes in and we do whatever it takes to help her be strong and less susceptible to sinusitis during the holiday season. I take her case and give her a dose of her constitutional remedy. I've only prescribed one remedy for her over all these years—*Natrum muriaticum*—and she has responded very well to it. Those who need this remedy may have a sinus infection with large amounts of watery discharge, dry, chapped lips, and canker sores, as Loren did. Her need to withdraw when not feeling well, her concern with perfection and neatness, and her overall sensitive nature also point to this remedy. Loren also had the typical *Natrum muriaticum* craving for salty foods and aversion to fat which helped to confirm the prescription of this remedy.

I'm happy to report that over the last many holiday seasons, Loren has not experienced full blown sinusitis. She has lowered her standards a bit on house cleanliness and feels better able to focus loving attention on her children.

If *Natrum muriaticum* is such a good remedy for Loren, one might wonder why she still got those sinus infections over the first years of our work together? In fact, Loren was moving in the direction of balance, towards a higher level of health. We do not look for overnight miracles or expect our patients never to get sick. If we can see incremental but steady improvement, especially in someone who has struggled for years, we are doing good work. In addition to helping shift the predisposition to sinus problems and addressing the particular symptoms, the homeopathic remedy gave Loren the resolve to make relevant lifestyle changes that encouraged and maintained health. She felt empowered to help herself by reducing her stress and doing the things she knew would help her feel better. Would I have preferred for her to never have another sinus infection after our work began? Sure. But I also appreciate the process of healing and realize that it takes time to shift patterns and create new ones.

Each year, from November through February, I ask Loren to follow the natural medicine protocol below. These dosages were tailored for her and her particular situation and are offered here only as a reflection of that prescription. After the holidays are over, she tapers off all but the first two vitamins:

- High potency multiple vitamin
- B complex vitamin, 50 mg once a day
- Vitamin C, 1000mg, twice a day, to help support immune function, decrease swelling in the sinus area, and protect her from environmental exposure to illness

- Bromelain, 500 mg three times a day, derived from pineapple, this supplement helps to thin mucus and decrease swelling and inflammation
- Bioflavonoids, 500 mg, three times a day. This supplement has an anti-histamine effect by stabilizing mast cell membranes

I also encourage Loren to switch from caffeinated beverages to herbal teas such as chamomile that have a calming effect. Each year, we revisit her commitment to exercise and I impress upon her the importance, especially during these months, of sticking with her walking program as a way to counter stress, clear her mind, and get her circulation going—all of which support proper immune function.

Though meant to be a joy filled time of year, the holiday season has taken on the unfortunate role of stressing many people out and triggering illness. Using constitutional homeopathy along with some tried and true naturopathic protocols to support health, there is a way to help reclaim the holidays as a fulfilling and satisfying way to start the New Year.

The Heart of the Matter: Homeopathy Helps with an Irregular Heartbeat

When Abigail first came to see me for atrial fibrillation—an irregular heart rhythm—I was uncertain about whether to treat her. As the central organ of circulation that works for most of us with utter predictability and reliability, the heart is also subject to sudden turns of events. Some, as we all know, can be life threatening. I wanted to first review her cardiac workup and have the support of her cardiologist. And I wanted to take extra special care to understand her underlying family history and the history of her current problem, as I would for anyone who came to see me for such a serious condition.

Abigail was distraught about her diagnosis. Her doctors were urging her to take anti-arrythmia and anti-anxiety drugs, but she was concerned about the side effects, since she'd had bad experiences with conventional medications in the past. She was hoping a homeopathic remedy might help instead.

I had seen Abigail on and off as a patient for twenty years, but it had been six years since her last visit. Her past list of complaints had included chronic urinary tract infections, dry and irritated skin, and a significant set of family issues that were exacerbated by and probably also contributed to anxiety, low self-esteem, and insecurity. She had done well with the homeopathic remedies *Staphysagria* and *Silicea* at different times in her life.

The first thing one would notice about Abigail was her diminutive size. She had always been small boned, but when she came to see me this time in the fall of 2005, she seemed to be slipping away. At 4 feet 11 inches and 90 pounds, she took up very little space. Her skin was close to transparent, pulled taught over the outline of her prominent jaw. Her attire was what I would call 'perfect casual'—meaning neither fancy nor expensive but put together with an eye toward exact size, color choice and accessories. Her hair was pure white now and cut in a flattering bob that gave a carefree feeling to this otherwise highly strung, sixty year old, retired office manager.

Abigail's large, wide-opened eyes were brown and cool, and her smile never quite reached them. Her voice was a bit wavering and quiet, but her specific word choice to describe her symptoms and her current life situation were painstakingly exact. Her effort to tell me accurately and faithfully precisely how she felt was nothing short of heroic. On a day when I had more patients or less patience, I might find a visit with Abigail trying.

Abigail told me that with the exception of some dry skin, her body and spirits had been good these last six years. Her three adult children were settled and doing well, and her new marriage to a man a few years older was a source of terrific support and pride. After years in a stressful and difficult relationship, this change was welcome.

About a month before our visit, however, Abigail had begun to experience irregular heartbeats, especially at night. Perhaps because she was so thin, or more likely because she was very well tuned in to her own body through regular exercise and weekly yoga classes, she was immediately aware that something was amiss in the region of her heart. After visits to her primary care physician and a cardiologist, Abigail was diagnosed with atrial fibrillation.

Atrial fibrillation is an irregular heartbeat that begins in the top portions of the heart. A problem with the electrical system creates a kind of shudder, which interferes with the normal rhythm of cardiac pumping. Atrial fibrillation can put a patient more at risk for stroke because blood may collect in the heart and form clots that can be pumped out into the arteries. This can also cause a heart attack.

Many things can cause atrial fibrillation such as high blood pressure, history of heart attack or other heart conditions, lung illnesses, hyperthyroidism, excessive intake of alcohol or marijuana, or overuse of stimulants like caffeine or nicotine. For some people, however, there is no known reason why atrial fibrillation begins.

The most common symptoms of atrial fibrillation are light headedness, shortness of breath, fatigue, palpitations, pain in the chest and fainting.

An electrocardiogram or EKG, which tests the electrical system of the heart, helps a doctor to diagnose atrial fibrillation. An echocardiogram gives additional information about how the heart is pumping and what state the patient's valves are in.

Conventional medical treatments depend on the patient's symptoms, the reason for the atrial fibrillation (if known), and other risks the patient may have for stroke. Treatments may include cardioversion, where a small electrical shock is given to the heart to stimulate it back to a more normal rhythm, and/or anti-arrhythmia drugs to attempt to bring the heart back to its normal rhythm. Many patients are also placed on blood thinners or aspirin to help reduce the risk of stroke. If cardioversion and medication do not work, doctors may recommend cardiac ablation, a procedure where small sections of the heart are destroyed thereby forming scar tissue to interrupt the irregular heartbeat. A pacemaker may be needed afterward to recreate normal rhythm.

Or .... the patient might find their way to a homeopath! In my experience over the past two decades, I have found homeopathic treatment to be helpful in many patients with atrial fibrillation. I have had to refer some patients for more invasive conventional procedures when homeopathy did not help them. But I have also had patients come to me after procedures like cardioversion or anti-arrythmics didn't work or didn't give lasting results, and over time, homeopathic remedies have offered them a welcome reprieve from atrial fibrillation.

With all my patients, I aim to understand the whole person; I take the case, striving to see the atrial fibrillation in the context of the person's overall physical, mental and emotional health. There certainly are homeopathic medicines that tend to be used more frequently for people with heart problems, but I do not limit myself to those medicines. I cast my net wide, trying to grasp all elements of the person's life so that I can best find a remedy that will help the whole person.

Once I give a remedy and have allowed it time to act, I assess its overall impact on the patient. Of course, I want to see that the atrial fibrillation has been less frequent, less intense, and/or shorter in duration with each episode, but more than that, I want to see that other things that limit the patient have also improved. This might include better digestion and sleep, or less anxiety and depression, depending on the individual. And for all patients, I want to see improved focus and energy.

Abigail described her atrial fibrillation as a 'sort of thumping' in her chest, which was worse at night. It was very distracting and greatly impacted her ability to sleep. It happened most every night and sometimes persisted through the morning. With less sleep, she was tired and more likely to feel her symptoms. So, as you can see, she was caught in a cycle of worsening atrial fibrillation that was leading to strong symptoms of anxiety. Her anxiety was definitely worse at night in bed, but it extended throughout the day as well. She wondered if she would die from this; she wondered why this was happening to her, especially now, at this time in her life when things were finally going well. She worried about her heart, her health in general, her husband's health, her children, an upcoming event—anything was fair game. She felt the anxiety in her stomach or in her chest or all over, and it did seem to make the atrial fibrillation worse.

When the atrial fibrillation really got going, she felt light-headed and off balance. She did not have any history of cardiac issues and had taken good care of her physical body over the years.

Abigail was very chilly, her extremities in particular. She had begun to wear earmuffs and gloves, though we were barely into a not-very-chilly autumn, and to use a heating blanket to warm her bed (turning it off before climbing in). Abigail especially felt cold in her back; she was always aware of any breeze or moving air and would often sit in a chair wrapped in an afghan to keep the cold from getting to her back. She perspired profusely especially on her head, hands and feet. She had always had a propensity for getting swollen glands; over the years they'd hardened, leaving chains of small knotty nodes under her jaw.

Her appetite was off; especially when she was having the atrial fibrillation, she did not particularly want to eat. She had always had a tendency towards constipation, going several days between bowel movements. It was as if she just didn't have the energy to push the stool out. She often bloated up and felt like her abdomen was swollen in the day leading up to a bowel movement.

She had some shortness of breath, which she attributed to being out of shape, due to not exerting herself as it seemed to aggravate her atrial fibrillation. Her fatigue was marked and worsening from the lack of sleep, the lack of exercise and the anxiety. She just wanted to lie down and rest all the time.

Abigail was careful in her speech—tentative is the word that comes to mind—and also painfully self-effacing (recall the *Staphysagria* prescription); I found myself speaking in a lower and lower voice and more slowly, too, so as not to overwhelm her. I asked my questions, she gave me her clearly thought-out answers. There was virtually no chitchat.

When I feel myself shifting in response to the way a patient presents, I know that likely I should be paying attention as to why. Part of this is common sense, any moderately sensitive person would do the same. I also use it to help me better understand the patient.

Abigail told me that her patient, caring husband would listen to her at great length and seemed to really appreciate her thoughtful care and careful thought. They soon would be moving to a warm island community (should help any condition), and making plans and anticipating the monumental changes were very stressful for Abigail. However, they were working together and trying to take it one step at a time.

Abigail was as organized as they come. As always, she brought me her medical records in perfect order, three-hole punched in a binder with typed labels on the dividers, and clearly marked folders for certain documents she did not want to put holes in. This made my review of her recent lab work and studies easy and straightforward, something I always appreciated about Abigail.

Of course, I also realized that Abigail's organized manner was a characteristic that could help point to a particular homeopathic remedy. With any such characteristic of a patient's temperament, I need to perceive why the person is like that—why she is so organized and conscientious, why being like that is important to her. Different 'remedy types' are careful and conscientious for different reasons. For instance, people who benefit from *Baryta carbonica* will be conscientious because they are deeply insecure; if they can have everything look 'together,' perhaps no one will be able to tell. *Calcarea carbonica* types are irritated by things out of place; many people needing this remedy will feel almost relaxed as they tidy up and organize possessions, papers or a particular area, like the fridge or the CD collection or the kids' toys. *Nux vomica* patients will want order and a specific place for everything because they have issues with control and want things their way and only their way.

It's important to remember that it is not just the symptom or the person's temperament that has meaning or value to the homeopath. Rather, everything we are told by the patient or that we observe during the case taking is context dependent; understanding what causes the patient to be that way and what they may derive from that tendency or symptom will help lead us to a prescription that can help the whole patient, including their chief complaint.

For Abigail, her need to be organized stemmed from deep anxieties that drove her to stick to the rules. She had a kind of rigidity to her life, and she put undue pressure on herself to adhere to what she deemed to be correct. Indeed, I believe her conscientious speech was another example of this—wanting to get it 'just right.' She needed to create strict order out of any chaos and build a life where surprises and unpredictable things would be less likely to happen. Even so, if a strong willed or strong minded person with a clear opinion and a loud voice came along, she would acquiesce. She did not like discord and avoided it at all cost.

My initial inclination in choosing a homeopathic remedy for Abigail was to head right back to the *Silicea* because it had helped her in the past, and she had retained many of her *Silicea* qualities especially in the emotional realm (her conscientiousness) and in her physical general symptoms (her tendency to be chilly, especially in the extremities, and her need to wrap up, as well as her easy perspiration). So I repeated the *Silicea* 200c and asked her to return in three weeks.

Unfortunately, when she returned, I learned that the remedy had no effect on her atrial fibrillation or her anxiety, and little to no effect on anything else, although perhaps she was moving her bowels a tad better. I assessed the *Silicea* as an incorrect prescription and went to work finding a remedy that was better suited to her with her current complaints.

As I studied Abigail's case, I noticed a remedy coming through the repertorization that I have not often prescribed: *Kalium silicatum*. Those who need one of the *Kalium* salts on a constitutional level (for example, *Kalium carbonicum, Kalium nitricum,* etc.) typically share common *Kalium* symptoms: needing a lot of structure and doing well with rules, while being wracked with anxiety and worry. But since *Kalium silicata* also has a *Silicea* component, *Kalium silicata's* indications also capture the symptoms of this patient that were so helped by *Silicea* in the past, such as her weakness, constipation and chilliness. In addition, it was as if Abigail were wasting away, and this is a kind of emaciation that *Kalium silicatum* is known for. She had this insidious weakness and fatigue, but like any good *Kalium* person, she forced herself to get up and work, to take care of business and keep going, owed in great part to her strong sense of duty.

I prescribed *Kalium silicatum* 12c, one pellet, once a day, and asked her to return to me in a month. I had felt comfortable giving Abigail *Silicea* in a higher potency (200c) since she had done well with it before; but I decided on a low potency with repeated doses for *Kalium silicatum* because Abigail had a kind of fragility about her.

Abigail phoned me a week after she began taking the *Kalium silicatum*. She said she felt better overall, her fatigue had lessened and her energy was higher, and she was sleeping better. She had not had any strong symptoms of the atrial fibrillation for that week—which was quite a marked improvement—though she still felt a sort of uneasiness in the region of her heart. She just wanted me to know that she thought we were on the right track.

That was a very heartening phone call to receive as I knew that if she had not gotten results soon, her cardiologist would surely be requiring her to try stronger conventional measures; I noted this in her chart and looked forward to seeing her in the office a month later. When she returned, the improvements had persisted. She had had just two nights of atrial fibrillation, over the whole month—quite a dramatic shift from before taking *Kalium silicatum* when she was experiencing it nightly and sometimes into the day. Her sleep was better, she felt less stressed out. She continued to struggle with constipation and being chilly. I decided to keep her on the *Kalium silicatum*12c daily for a while, mostly because she was continuing to improve and I did not want to rock the boat.

In has been more than two years now since Abigail started treatment to address atrial fibrillation, and she is very pleased with the results. In these two years, she has had a few weeks where the atrial fibrillation seemed to crop up again just a bit, especially during times of great stress, but never to the degree she had been experiencing it before homeopathic treatment. I have given her *Kalium silicatum* in higher potency as the need arises. Over this time, she has also gotten better at recognizing the atrial fibrillation as a symptom that is related to her stress, and instead of escalating into severe anxiety, she will take a deep breath and try to figure out how to cut the stress down. She is ever grateful to homeopathy for once again helping her find a better place of balance.

So with Abigail, I re-learned the lesson that treating atrial fibrillation with homeopathy is a worthwhile endeavor. Each time I have a success treating someone with a cardiac condition, I feel more inspired to treat others. With our aging population, I should have no shortage of opportunities!

The Man Who Married His Job: A Case of Chronic Heartburn and Acid Reflux

When 52 year old Harold first came to see me some years ago, his chief complaint of gastroesophageal reflux (GERD) was getting him down. His stomach acid would sometimes flow backward (or reflux) into his esophagus. Harold's symptoms had begun years before as mild heartburn and had progressively worsened to the point of constant irritation in his esophagus and a bad taste in his mouth. He worried about what and how to eat and about how the GERD might put him at risk or lead him to other gastrointestinal problems, like peptic ulcer or esophageal cancer.

Harold told me that he had suffered from heartburn most of his adult life. It would come on if he ate very spicy foods or if he lay down after eating a big meal. But in the last two years, Harold had been under unusual stress at home and at work, and heartburn had become an almost constant annoyance—regardless of what food he ate or what he did after meals. Harold felt heat and burning in his upper chest; he battled a sour taste in his mouth and would daily regurgitate food by the mouthful. To avoid the problem, he would often skip eating.

In the past year, Harold had gone through a difficult divorce, and at work, things had been extremely stressful too. After many years at the helm of his own consulting firm doing work he loved, Harold had been blindsided by problems with the bookkeeping and dishonest employees. He was upset that this had happened right under his nose and he felt responsible for the monies lost. He was also disappointed in himself, knowing that he had taken out his work frustrations on his family and ex-wife. As he spoke, however, it was clear to me that Harold had put most of these emotional issues behind him; he was now strongly focused on trying to find help for his worsening reflux condition.

Harold's doctors had prescribed several conventional acid-blocking or acid-inhibiting medications in succession. The drugs had taken the edge off his symptoms, but his current prescription seemed to be working less and less effectively. Harold didn't like the way it made him feel, nor did he like the idea of having to take such a drug for the long term. He also understood that many of these drugs could cause problems down the road by interfering with stomach acid production, transit time of food through the gastrointestinal tract, and the early line of defense against germs that stomach acids provide.

Harold was determined to beat his GERD naturally. "I'm ready to do whatever you suggest," he said briskly. A small, compact man, Harold was alert, energetic, efficient—and all business. He reported his symptoms with precision and clarity. He was no-nonsense all the way through our interview and took ample notes on my recommendations.

I always ask patients with GERD about other illnesses they may have and especially about other medications they may be taking, since many conventional medications cause GERD (for example, calcium channel blockers, beta-2 agonists, Diazepam and opioid analgesics). Harold was not taking any of these medications, and a review of his health history and bodily systems found him to be quite healthy, except for the GERD. He did not suffer from headaches, common winter illnesses or allergies; his skin was clear and his urinary tract functioned well. He had a tendency to get constipated especially if he traveled for work, which he addressed by taking a fiber supplement when on the road. He was not particularly thirsty, but he did want and need a few cups of green tea each morning. (He had other food cravings and aversions, but I did not put much weight on these symptoms when selecting a homeopathic remedy because he had over-analyzed them, due to the nature of his chief complaint).

Harold was chilly by nature and considered himself a morning person. He complained of some insomnia, especially of late, with his business woes. He would wake at night, worried and anxious, and then get out of bed and check his email or write himself notes about the upcoming day.

Harold said he was quick tempered and irritable by nature, but he would get over things just as quickly, and faster than most people. He believed he was a good boss, demanding but also able to appreciate a job well done. A self-described workaholic, he got along well with people but didn't have many friends. "My ex-wife often complained that I was married to the job more than to her ... that I gave more time and attention to the office than I ever gave to her," he admitted. In effect, that is why his marriage ended; his wife felt that she was never a priority to him. As Harold shared these reflections during our interview, he did not deny any of them.

For newer homeopathic practitioners, every case must be studied and pored over, but as we gain experience with patients and with remedies, it can at times be quite easy to make a good and effective remedy choice. I did not need to repertorize Harold's symptoms or study my *materia medica* to choose a remedy. It was a clear 'pattern recognition' case; there were enough chief complaint, physical general, and mental-emotional symptoms to lead me directly to the remedy *Nux vomica*.

To quote Boericke in his *materia medica*: "*Nux* is pre-eminently the remedy for many of the conditions incident to modern life. The typical *Nux* patient is rather thin, spare, quick, active, nervous, and irritable. He does a good deal of mental work; has mental strains and leads a sedentary life, found in prolonged office work, over study, and close application to business, with its cares and anxieties." Boericke continues that *Nux vomica* is "especially adapted to digestive disturbances." Harold's GERD symptoms, sour taste in his mouth, constipation, insomnia, chilliness and need for stimulants (tea) are also very typical *Nux vomica* symptoms.

I gave Harold one dose of *Nux vomica* 200c and, as I do with all my patients, told him what I would expect with this remedy and the rest of the plan. I thought the GERD would lessen in intensity and that, on some days, he would be symptom-free. I hoped the remedy might also take the edge off the way he experienced the stress and worry in his life. I recommended that he not stop his current allopathic prescription drug but rather to wait and see how he did over the course of the next six weeks. If he felt better, we would then start to slowly decrease his medication.

With a complaint like GERD, I depend on homeopathy to help address the underlying tendency to develop the problem in the first place, but I also use other natural medicine treatments and lifestyle modification approaches to good effect. See page 201 that outlines the recommendations I drew up for Harold.

When Harold returned six weeks later, he greeted me with a hearty handshake and a big smile. In that moment, I knew we had found a good plan for him. "The first thing to go was that bad taste in my mouth," he reported. "And in the very first week, I began to sleep better, too." The reflux was still with him, but as I had predicted, it was less intense and interspersed with symptom-free days.

Against my recommendations, Harold had discontinued his allopathic medicine. I do not support this kind of action; I like to move slowly in ways that are not shocking to the system, but some patients have their own ideas, and since Harold's health did seem to be moving in the right direction, there was little I could say. I encouraged Harold to stick with our original plan, and I did not repeat the *Nux vomica* at that time.

Four years later, Harold continued to do well. Two or three times a year he will show up or call and ask for another dose of *Nux vomica*. He has cut back on the rest of his natural medicine GERD supplements, but keeps them handy in case he feels a return of any of his old symptoms.

In addition to prescribing the indicated constitutional homeopathic remedy for a patient with heartburn or gastroesophageal reflux problems, I typically recommend the following supportive measures, as I did for Harold.

DGL, or deglycyrrhizinated licorice is derived from the herb licorice, but the part of the plant that tends to raise blood pressure has been removed. It works to help soothe, nourish and support healthy mucus membrane linings of the esophagus, stomach and intestine. Dose: one capsule before each meal. On a day when symptoms are particularly strong, another capsule may be taken at bedtime.

Slippery Elm lozenges help soothe the lining of the upper respiratory and gastrointestinal tracts. Lozenges can be taken liberally throughout the day, especially when feeling stressed out and the gastrointestinal tract seems to be taking the brunt of it.

Slippery Elm or Marshmallow Root Tea work at soothing and supporting the lining as described above. They are good to keep handy and use at least one to two times a day. I also like Throat Coat tea by Traditional Medicinals, which includes slippery elm and other herbs.

The minerals Zinc and copper help to rebuild the proper lining of the mucus membranes of the upper respiratory tract.

Dose: a ratio of 15 mg of Zinc to 1 to 2 mg of copper would be considered one daily dose.

Lifestyle changes recommended include:

- Drink as little as possible (preferably nothing) with meals. Water should be consumed between meals.
- Chew food really well. This may sound obvious but the goal is to give food a bit of a head start by fully using the digestive enzymes present in saliva.
- The largest meal should be at lunchtime or in the late afternoon.
- Take a short walk after eating. Don't lie down!
- Make healthy stress reduction part of daily life. I support any such activities that are enjoyable for the individual (for example exercising, painting, listening to music, meditating, gardening, woodworking, writing, etc.).

Forbes magazine often lists the top ten best selling drugs in the world. In recent times, coming in at number three was Nexium®, and at number nine, Prevacid®. With such rampant use, these heartburn drugs are big money makers for the pharmaceutical companies and are not cheap for the buyers. When considering one's treatment options, it seems only logical to give homeopathy and other effective, more affordable natural medicine approaches a chance. Harold was certainly convinced after his experience—as have been many satisfied patients who've taken this route.

Never Well Since the Flu

Elaine first came to see me in the fall of 1992. She had been sick for eight years, she said, ever since a bad case of the flu. In the winter of 1985 she had had the worst case of flu imaginable: fever, body aches, sore throat, utter exhaustion and seemingly endless amounts of mucus. She'd spent weeks in bed, trying many over-the-counter and home remedies to little avail. She crawled her way back to functionality, but ever since that time she had been plagued with numerous health problems.

I have more than a few patients who have developed chronic complaints after a bout with the flu. In the course of their healing via homeopathy, some of these patients go back through a flu-like episode; others do not. Sometimes their current symptoms are similar to those that they had when they had the flu—and sometimes not. In Elaine's case, her symptoms were mostly different from the symptoms she had with her original flu.

Elaine said she had a constant, chronic, low grade sinus infection, terribly bad breath, frequent headaches, a hoarse voice and zero energy. She told me that she used to be an energetic and upbeat person but that since her bad case of the flu, she had lost much of her enthusiasm for life. She is a stay-at-home mom who used to love the job. Now she felt unable to offer the creative touch to homemaking or motherhood. She merely got through the day, feeding and clothing her three children.

As any homeopath would, I asked her to describe each of her above mentioned complaints so that I could understand how she experienced them. It is not enough for the homeopath to hear 'sinusitis.' We must know: Which side? What does the pain feel like (burning, stabbing, pressing)? Is there anything that makes the pain better (pressure, hot application, cold application)? Or is there anything that makes the pain worse (going outdoors, motion, stooping, etc.)? There is no such thing as a simple symptom to the homeopath—we seek to understand each and every symptom in all its glory. New patients sometimes are at a loss for answers to some of our questions, but as they get the hang of visiting their homeopath, they learn what kind of information is not only valued, but essential.

After gleaning that information from Elaine about her main complaints, I also wanted to see her physical symptoms in the context of the rest of her overall health; I needed to understand about her digestion, urination, sleep, musculoskeletal system, respiration, skin, menstrual cycle, etc. This 'review of systems' offers the homeopath a wonderful opportunity to scan through the person's health history, to turn up any problem areas that may have gone unremembered by the patient.

As it turned out, Elaine had had a terrible problem with constipation since her bout with the flu; she could go days without a bowel movement, and there was often mucus in her stool. In addition, she complained of calluses on her feet, and her nails broke and chipped with little provocation. Her hair was thin, fell out freely, and she described it as 'limp and lackluster.'

The homeopath also seeks to know the general physical aspects of their patient. Elaine was very chilly, wore a hat except in summer, and though she was so cold, she sweat easily, especially on her feet. She had no particular food cravings or aversions, but was partial year round to warm drinks.

As I moved through her interview, I observed Elaine to be a quiet, reserved woman with a carefulness about her. She chose her words intentionally and did not embellish her answers. She was soft spoken and receding in her manner. I mentioned this observation and she agreed, "Yes, I don't take up much space in my family, I'm the peacemaker, I don't like discord. I am insecure and often feel inferior to those around me. I apologize constantly, even if it's not my fault."

Since her bout with the flu, her whole demeanor had shifted, she told me. She felt overly dependent on her husband, which made her feel weak and unable to fend for herself. She often became overwhelmed with the role of taking care of the children and keeping house.

I felt I had a good homeopathic remedy for her, a remedy that could help address the physical concerns she was experiencing since she'd had the flu—but also a remedy that could help strengthen her from within, to shore up her spirits and enable her to embrace life, her family, and her own interests more fully.

I prescribed the remedy *Silicea* based on the type of sinusitis she suffered. She had thick mucus which was difficult to dislodge, she experienced pinpoint pains to the face, and she felt better with warm applications and warm drinks. Also reminiscent of *Silicea* were the bad breath and the chronic constipation—without the urge to go and with a sense of a lump in her rectum —which she had endured for years. These physical discomforts were woven together in my analysis with her yielding, conscientious nature and her self-esteem issues, leading me to *Silicea* as a constitutional remedy. It should be noted that any remedy can be used to treat a person who has never been well since a flu—the whole person must be considered, with all of their symptomatology.

I asked Elaine to return six weeks later. I also asked her to call me if she became ill during that time so that together we might try to help her fight off any acute illness.

Sure enough, she returned six weeks later, elated and bursting with gratitude—she felt she was 'back.' This is a wonderful report to a homeopath's ears. When patients say that they feel they are 'back to their old selves,' we know they are moving in the right direction. Even if some of Elaine's physical symptoms had not gone away—and most of them had—I would've stuck with this remedy after a good report like that, trusting that she was on the healing path and her vital force would continue the work it had begun.

Indeed, I did not give her another dose of *Silicea* until some eight months later when she seemed to have relapsed a bit the first inkling of that was a return of the constipation.

I have seen Elaine periodically over the last decade, through the many trials and challenges that life offers up. Sometimes she gets another dose of *Silicea*, sometimes we talk about diet and exercise or particular home remedies she might try. She remains thankful and even incredulous that those little pills could finally take a hold of that old flu and put it where it belonged.

From Nursing to Hot Flashes: A Middle-aged Mom's Dilemma

When Georgia came to see me a few years ago, she was a 48 year old mother of a delightful two year old. She had not set out to become a parent in her mid-forties, but that is how her life had unfolded. Now, like many other women her age, she was facing the demands of a capricious toddler while being challenged by the unpredictability of her own body and mind during the years of perimenopause. It seemed an unfair coupling, to go straight from the emotional upheavals that can accompany nursing to the mood shifts associated with menopause—from sleepless nights due to a waking baby, to interrupted sleep due to hot flashes and hormonal changes.

More and more women who opt to have children later in life are facing this same dilemma: no break between having and raising small children and going through menopause. On either side of the equation, homeopathy can help with the physical, mental and emotional symptoms that some women face when going through menopause.

The hormonal shifts of the perimenopausal years are a kind of stress on the female system. Women react to these shifts in hormones with symptoms, just as they would to other kinds of stressors. It is the homeopath's job to take a woman's symptoms and find a remedy to match—a remedy that will help to reduce the intensity, severity and duration of these troubling complaints. The longer range issues related to osteoporosis and heart disease, two physical ailments that increase in the female population after menopause, can also be addressed with homeopathy as well as with other gentle, effective natural medicine. Below, I will share one woman's story of the more acute challenges of menopause.

Georgia's main complaints were terrible mood swings with irritability, as well as persistent and constant hot flashes. That she was snapping at her co-workers, husband, daughter, and even the dog, was not new for her—she had always had the tendency to be snappish during the week before her menses. That she was now irritable all the time and snapping as a first response—this was new. Georgia was embarrassingly aware of how her short temper and negative energy were affecting everyone around her, most especially her young daughter who seemed to be almost cowering around her mother. Anything could set Georgia off: burning a piece of toast, a cluttery mess in the house, her husband being a bit late, the fallibility of a colleague. She would murmur under her breath, snarl and then snap. She would be brusque and rude around the house. She would yell and mean it. To her credit, Georgia would get over these outbursts quickly, would apologize and move on. But she felt she was leaving a wake of anger in her path.

Add to that the fact that she was having intense and long lasting hot flashes that left her hot, sweaty and cranky. They were unpredictable and came on suddenly, worse at night and fairly constant throughout the month. She was going into her eighth or ninth month of hot flashes; she had tried vitamin E and some herbal hormone support tablets to no avail. She would feel warmth begin in her abdomen and spread quickly up through her torso and on to her face. Her complexion would go from a basic paleness to bright red with each flash; indeed I saw this several times during our interview. Georgia had learned, like many others, to dress in layers and be prepared to pull off sweaters and open collars.

As if this was not enough, Georgia had begun bleeding terribly with each menstrual cycle. Though her cycles were still fairly regular, her bleeding pattern had shifted dramatically. Her annual gynecological exam had been normal, with no evidence of fibroids or other problems. That said, she was bleeding much more heavily than at other times in her life and for more days. She would be exhausted by the end of her cycle, although she was not anemic. Now, along with an overstuffed diaper bag, Georgia felt she needed to pack a change of clothes for herself, in case she had an accident. The blood itself was bright red, without clots and seemed to flow freely through the day and night.

The migraine headaches that Georgia had suffered most of her life were still with her and still worse before her menstrual cycle. She would have the occasional migraine during the month, but would predictably have one before each and every period. She was looking forward to the cessation of her periods, with the hope that it would put an end to these seemingly hormonal headaches. The nature of the headache was bursting; a feeling of pressure would build up in her head as the days led up to her menstrual flow. Once the bleeding began, she would feel some relief.

In all, Georgia was exhausted. She was exhausted from running after a two year old, exhausted from the demands of her full time job as a secretary, and exhausted by the constant hot flashes and heavy menstrual flow. She also felt like she had gone right from 'milk brain,' the mildly pleasant state of not being as mentally agile during the months of nursing, to becoming a 'space shot.' She would forget why she came into a room or a store, would lose thoughts mid-sentence, and would feel tongue-tied. In what she affectionately called her 'previous life,' her sharp mind and sure articulateness were amongst her strongest attributes.

So, Georgia was dealing with symptoms that she had suffered with for much of her adult life—premenstrual irritability and headaches—on top of symptoms of menopause—constant, rather unrelenting irritability, hot flashes, weariness, poor concentration, and excess bleeding with her periods. Indeed, the added pressures and expectations of motherhood and running a busy household along with the hormonal shifts of menopause were wreaking havoc on Georgia's otherwise happy life.

When choosing a remedy for Georgia, I wanted one whose indications had some energy and intensity to them. Conversely, I also wanted a remedy that could address the exhausted and wiped out side of Georgia. The remedies that came through repertorization of her symptoms were: *Belladonna, Calcarea carbonica, Lachesis, Phosphorus* and *Sulphur.*

Because *Lachesis* is an often used remedy for women during the change of life and because its symptoms tend to be intense, I considered it for Georgia. The fact that she was so much relieved at the beginning of her menstrual flow certainly fit the *Lachesis* profile. But Georgia lacked the characteristic jealous nature and the suspiciousness entirely, and she had no issues related to feelings of restriction around her abdomen or neck, as one might expect of a woman who needed *Lachesis*. Apart from her tendency towards irritability, her relationship with her husband was basically pretty sweet.

Instead, I choose *Belladonna* as it best matches the totality and intensity of Georgia's story. It covers the sudden onset and severity of her hot flashes, the sudden bursts of anger and quick resolution, and the excess bleeding of her menses, bright red and free flowing. Although *Belladonna* is often used by homeopaths and parents alike for acute illness, it must be remembered as a wonderful remedy for constitutional treatment as well. No homeopathic remedy can ever be strictly categorized as only for acute or only for chronic situations; we must remain open to whatever the best remedy is for the patient at any given time.

I gave Georgia one dose of *Belladonna* 200c in the office and asked her to return two months later. I wanted her to have at least two menstrual cycles to allow us to assess the efficacy of the remedy.

When she returned, this time with her toddler in tow, I became privy to much more than in the first interview. Georgia's daughter, brought in for the treatment of chronic earaches, was also a constitutional *Belladonna* patient. What a pair they were! Fiery, intense, bright eyed, full of energy and life! I could tell that when things were good, they were very good in that household, but when tempers flared, well, others best duck for cover!

Georgia reported that she had not had a migraine headache since she had taken the *Belladonna*. Her hot flashes were fewer in number and less severe. Her sleep had improved because she was having fewer hot flashes at night or was better able to sleep through them. Most importantly, she felt a calmness, a return to her ability to troubleshoot and handle problems as they arose. She was not so exhausted and was more patient with her daughter, and she was finding pleasure once again in the day-to-day running of a household. She felt more on the ball at work, less scatterbrained. Her menstrual period was still heavy with regard to flow.

In all, this was an excellent first follow-up, with widespread improvements; it appeared that the *Belladonna* was working.

Georgia was thrilled with the results and asked for 'more of that remedy.'

Not so fast, I said! A perfect way to ruin a perfect case would be to give more of the remedy when it was not needed. I told her she was doing great and would likely continue to do so. I asked her to return in another two months or to call before then if she felt her symptoms were worsening.

She called about a month later complaining that the hot flashes were getting worse again and she was starting to become irritable. We repeated the *Belladonna* 200c, and she again responded well with the irritability and hot flashes greatly diminishing. Over the course of that year she had *Belladonna* 1M two more times when it became indicated again, and she continued to do very well.

It was a year or so later that Georgia's periods ceased. She had more comfortably navigated the waters of menopause and had come out on the other side intact—a calmer, happier, healthier mother of an adorable preschooler.

Wear and Tear Arthritis —What Can be Done to Ease the Pain?

As a practicing licensed naturopathic physician, I've received many phone calls and emails from arthritis sufferers looking for answers. With anti-inflammatory drugs like Vioxx®, Celebrex®, Naproxen® and Bextra® under scrutiny or pulled from the market, patients far and wide are wondering if gentler, effective approaches might exist in the world of complementary and alternative medicine (CAM). Osteoarthritis sufferers do have some CAM treatment options, which I'll discuss below.

Anyone considering beginning a new treatment protocol, however, should do so under the guidance of his or her local physician. In addition, this chapter addresses osteoarthritis *only*. Rheumatoid arthritis, psoriatic arthritis, gout and other joint diseases require different treatment approaches.

Osteoarthritis or degenerative joint disease is common. In the US, it's estimated that more than 80 percent of people over age 50 have it to some degree. The joints that do the most work— knees, hips, back and hands—are most often affected. Cartilage normally cushions the ends of bones within a joint; but osteoarthritis leads to breakdown of cartilage and bones rubbing against each other. Typical symptoms are morning stiffness, painful swollen joints, reduced range of motion and possible deformation of the joints. Normal wear and tear on the body is enough to cause problems, especially for those with a family history of arthritis or other risk factors. Things that can make arthritis worse include food allergies, mineral deposits in the joints, past injury to the area, poor diet, stress, excess weight (adds stress to the weight bearing joints), hormone imbalance and changes in barometric pressure.

Like all medicine, CAM recommendations work best when applied as soon as possible after diagnosis. Prognosis depends on the severity of the arthritis, the length of time someone has had it, tissue changes that have occurred, simultaneous medical conditions (both physical and emotional), and the person's ability to carry out the treatment protocol.

Some CAM approaches (for example, certain herbs or supplements) work in a mechanistic way, by reducing inflammation and encouraging circulation. Other CAM approaches (like homeopathy or Chinese medicine) take an entirely different view of health and disease, with treatment plans individualized to the patient and how they experience their arthritis.

As a premier CAM approach, homeopathy has much to offer. I always look for an arthritis patient's constitutional homeopathic remedy—a remedy that will reduce inflammation and pain in the joint *as the person moves to a more balanced overall state of health.* I choose a remedy that addresses how the patient experiences their arthritis symptoms, what brings the pain on, what makes it better or worse, how it impacts their overall health, and whether any other symptoms arise when the joints are especially inflamed. I try to see how arthritis fits into their life and if there are elements in the mental or emotional sphere that might need attention.

It's quite common for a patient to see me for some health problem, and return after homeopathic treatment to report, "by the way Doc, not only is my indigestion (or asthma or PMS or...) better, but my joints are much better, too." The patient may not have even mentioned their arthritis in the initial consult. As a patient under constitutional treatment moves towards health, however, she will improve on many levels—physical, emotional and mental.

The following foods are known to have anti-inflammatory effects, so I suggest that my osteoarthritis patients add them to their diets.

- Foods high in essential fatty acids, like flax seed and cold water fish
- Fruits high in Bioflavonoids, like blueberries, raspberries, blackberries

- Foods high in the element sulfur, like asparagus, garlic, onions, cabbage
- Pineapple, as it contains the anti-inflammatory enzyme, Bromelain

I promote a diet high in vegetable fiber to keep the bowels moving and rid the body of that which it does not need. I also remind patients that eating meat tends to acidify the body, which can lead to more pain and inflammation.

Food allergies have been associated with arthritis and arthritis pain, but here's the catch—the most common offenders are foods that make up most typical American diets: dairy, wheat, eggs, citrus, refined sugars and eggs. So if you are someone who *would be willing to follow a more limited diet*, you should get tested for food allergies. After testing, it's important to work with a qualified nutritionist to come up with a diet and menu plan that incorporates the newfound information.

The supplements I recommend have been endorsed by clinical studies in peer-reviewed medical journals. They include: glucosamine sulfate, fish oil, low dose vitamin E, vitamin C and Bromelain. If needed, I will suggest adding digestive enzymes to improve digestion and support proper elimination. For some patients, I add a botanical medicine formula that includes herbs such as Ginger, alfalfa, turmeric and white willow, all of which contain anti-inflammatory capacities. Dosages and frequency depend on the patient's weight, other supplements or medications they might be taking, their level of pain, and their pain tolerance.

I often recommend simple hydrotherapy techniques that patients can do at home. For those with arthritis, the simplest is the hot bath with 1--2 cups of Epsom salt (magnesium sulfate) dissolved in the water, which helps to draw out inflammation.

Stress reduction techniques are another important component to the CAM approach to arthritis. Whether for you that means yoga, meditation, prayer, music, socializing, massage, reading, exercising or gardening, it is essential to build such activities into your daily life, as both a preventive and treatment measure.

A Patient Story of Recurring Hives

When Shelly came into my office for the first time, her bare arms were dotted with clusters of red, swollen, bumps—swaths of hives! Having successfully treated many cases of hives in my career, I had a strong feeling that I could help her. This 44 year old government worker and mother of two explained that she'd been suffering with angry, itchy eruptions for five years and was at her wit's end. The hives were interrupting her ability to work, to relax and to do things she enjoyed. They also greatly affected her sleep, which in turn influenced everything else in her life.

Though I never want my patients to suffer, I do find it helpful when their chief complaint is something like Shelly's that I can clearly see. The easiest people to treat successfully with homeopathy are those with clear, strong symptoms. It's also advantageous if these symptoms vary predictably and have definite modalities (that is have specific conditions that 'modify' the symptoms or make them better or worse, such as 'better from warmth' or 'worse from wet weather'). It became apparent soon into our consultation that Shelly's complaint of severe hives had all these characteristics—unambiguous symptoms, definite modalities and predictable variability—which made me all the more optimistic that I could help her with homeopathy.

Hives (also known as urticaria) are raised, reddish bumps or wheals on the skin that usually itch and sometimes burn or sting. Hives can vary in size from a few millimeters to a foot in diameter; they can be distinct or may grow together to form larger plaques. They generally arise in fast measure and occur in outbreaks that come and go. For some people, hives disappear just as quickly as they come, but for others, they linger. Most hives don't last longer than 24 hours, but sometimes they persist or reoccur on other parts of the body in cycles that last for weeks.

Most hive eruptions are thought to occur after contact with some sort of allergen, such as foods, drugs, food additives and preservatives, insects or pet dander. Hives can also be triggered by things like sun, heat, cold, pressure, and sometimes, infections. It is often easier to pinpoint the instigating factor in acute cases of hives than in chronic cases; for many people, no cause is ever determined. Those prone to hay fever and other allergies are typically more likely to get hives.

I have personally witnessed an increase in the occurrence of hives and in the intensity and duration of breakouts in the population. We are, in general, becoming a more allergic people; there are many theories as to why that is so, varying from children's lack of contact with simple dirt, to the overuse of antibacterial products, to the impact on our immune system from an environment that has become less than pristine. Hives are just one way such allergies manifest.

Luckily, homeopathy has much to offer these patients who often come to us for help when they are at the end of their rope. In addition to giving a well chosen homeopathic remedy, we homeopaths emphasize the importance of removing contact with the offending agent, if it is known. We also recommend applying cool compresses, keeping room temperatures cool, and removing tight-fitting garments.

Sometimes hives can develop into an emergency situation. If a patient experiences difficult breathing, severe vertigo, a tight feeling in the chest, or any swelling of the tongue, lips or face, they should go to the emergency room immediately. It's not that homeopathic remedies cannot also help at such moments, but we never want a loved one or a patient to be at risk.

Shelly explained to me that when she first began getting hives five years earlier, they would be small, perhaps the size of a quarter, mostly on the abdomen, and would go away on their own after some hours. In the first few years, the eruptions seemed to arise in the week or so before her menstrual period, were worse in the colder months, and had an affinity for the right side of the abdomen. Her family doctor prescribed Zyrtec®, an antihistamine, which seemed to help for a while, but soon afterwards, "the hives took on a life of their own," Shelly said. They grew larger, were itchier and were coming rapid-fire all month long. The Zyrtec® and other medications she tried didn't seem to be helping as much anymore.

Shelly had tried to figure out what was causing her hives by paying attention to her diet and environment but in the end could not arrive at any definitive answers. She noticed that when the hives were bad (larger, redder, more itchy), her thinking was impacted. She did not feel clear minded, could not make simple decisions, and felt overwhelmed. She also felt that she became unreasonably irritable and short tempered at home and at work.

As the years passed, Shelly's situation worsened. This earnest, forthcoming if somewhat insecure patient explained that she began to notice that her swallowing was more difficult whenever she had hives. Her breathing also began to be affected during severe outbreaks. In crisis, she would have to make a trip to the emergency room for help. Such trips were now starting to become almost routine, and she could count on at least one visit to the ER each month.

It was at this point that Shelly sought my care, feeling like her conventional medical treatment was not benefitting her in the long run. Although her ER visits greatly helped her get through the breathing crises, her daily medications did not seem to be preventing the outbreaks in the first place. She was also unhappy with the necessity of being on prednisone, a strong steroid medication, to control inflammation, and on other strong antihistamines that made her tired.

Besides the hives, Shelly had a lifelong tendency for digestive tract issues. She told me that she tended to have indigestion, gas, bloating, and constipation. She had had right sided ovarian cysts during her 30s, though she hadn't had any lately. She reported heavy menstrual flow due to a uterine fibroid. She and her gynecologist were keeping an eye on that, and she was not anemic from excessive blood loss. She also described a history of fibrocystic breast disease, worse in the right breast, that had gotten much better since she removed caffeine from her diet some ten years ago.

This graceful and quiet patient complained of always being chilly, with a cold feeling that was difficult to alleviate. She said that she did not know how she could survive without an electric blanket to warm up her bed at night, although she turned off the electricity once she climbed in. All of her symptoms, including the hives, were worse in winter.

Shelly craved sweets and ate them liberally even though she would feel worse when she ate them, especially mentally. Cloudy thinking coupled with irritability were common feelings for her, and they were exacerbated by eating her treats. Shelly generally lost energy in the late afternoon, just when she needed it most to get through the dinner hour with her family. She would get a few good hours of work in before bed, and she said she slept well on the nights when the hives weren't too bad.

When looking at a story like Shelly's and considering how to treat her with homeopathy, it can be tempting to zero in on those intense and clear hives symptoms and give a remedy just for that complaint, such as *Apis mellifica* or *Urtica urens* or *Rhus toxicodendron*. Indeed, there are times when a remedy like one of these with a narrower sphere of influence and a great affinity for skin reactions like hives will be indicated. That said, more often than not, my experience has shown that a remedy that addresses the whole person, including but not limited to the hives, has a broader and deeper acting effect.

Looking at Shelly, a woman with a long thin face and a long elegant neck, I could see that she carried her weight in the hip area and in her belly. This body type coupled with her digestive tract issues, her chilliness, her history of fibrocystic breasts and ovarian cysts both worse on the right side, her late afternoon energy slump, and her craving for sweets led me to a particular remedy. Her cloudy thinking and irritability, which were exacerbated during incidences of hives, also pointed to this remedy: *Lycopodium clavatum.*

I believed that this was Shelly's constitutional remedy because Shelly had reacted to the various stressors in her life in the same way over time, and her reactions were consistent with the indications for *Lycopodium.* Whether the stressors were discord in the family or money troubles, Shelly would respond in the same way—she would develop digestive tract problems and irritability. As she got older, she started getting new local symptoms (i.e., hives), but her personality, temperament and physical general qualities never shifted. And her new hives symptoms had the same modalities and concomitant symptoms that she'd had all along: irritability, cloudy thinking, worse in the cold, etc.

It can also be noted that the *materia medica* for *Lycopodium* does include hives, as well as many other sorts of skin manifestations. Whenever we have a remedy that has a very wide sphere of influence, such as this one, we can suspect that it will cover common symptoms like hives, especially when the patient's general symptoms and mental/emotional symptoms are consistent with the remedy's indications.

I prescribed *Lycopodium* in a 12c daily dose. I chose a low potency, repeated daily, because she was also taking conventional medications. Since I presumed that *Lycopodium* was Shelly's constitutional remedy that she might need to take for many years, starting with a low potency also gave me room to increase the strength of the dose over time.

In addition, I asked Shelly to take Vitamin C and Bioflavonoids. These natural products are aimed at stabilizing the mast cell membranes in the blood. Among their other jobs, mast cells are responsible for releasing histamine, the culprit in many allergic reactions. By strengthening the mast cell membrane, we can reduce the amount of histamine released. I asked Shelly not to change any of her other medications and to return to see me in six weeks.

Shelly came into my office six weeks later with a big smile on her face, and I noticed that her bare arms looked almost normal again. She reported that she'd had fewer outbreaks of hives in the last six weeks, and those that she'd had were less severe. The eruptions didn't last as long and seemed to be smaller. What pleased Shelly the most was that she hadn't had any swallowing or breathing problems, and she'd not needed to go to the emergency room in crisis. I decided that things were going well and asked her to continue to take *Lycopodium* 12c once a day along with the other supplements.

When Shelly returned to see me two months later, she reported that the first month she'd continued to do well, but in the last three weeks, she seemed somewhat worse. I decided to stick with *Lycopodium* once a day but to increase the potency to 30c. We also decided that she would work with her family doctor on trying to slowly decrease her conventional medication.

Over the ensuing year, Shelly and I continued to work closely together, adjusting her dose as needed, and she eventually found that she could take a dose of *Lycopodium* 30c about once every 2–3 weeks and be relatively hive-free, even during winter.

My experience has shown that a remedy that addresses the whole person, including but not limited to the hives, has a broader and deeper acting effect.

Since that time, five years ago, I occasionally hear from Shelly, when she calls about one of her children. Her hives are mostly a thing of the past. Infrequently, she will get a skin eruption now but she never has any difficulties with swallowing or breathing. When she does get a mild hive outbreak, she takes a dose of *Lycopodium* 30c and that seems to take care of it. She no longer needs the strong conventional anti-histamines or steroids that she used to take, but she keeps her arsenal of pharmaceuticals on hand just in case of an emergency. On the other side of her medicine cabinet is her short line of bottles of *Lycopodium* 12c, 30c, and 200c. She calls me when she feels she needs to, but mostly she does not take the *Lycopodium* anymore and does not suffer from hives.

Shelly's long standing digestive troubles have improved greatly as well, and her overall energy level is higher. She is back to her weekly racquetball games, which she had avoided for months at a time during her years of hives. This alone has given her great satisfaction. She is happy to have her energy and focus back, and to no longer be held captive by the random effects of increasingly powerful hives.

When a patient comes in with clear, strong symptoms and definite modalities, I am optimistic about offering them help with homeopathic treatment. Their vital force is engaged and stimulated and putting out strong signals that point to a remedy. Especially in these situations, I encourage homeopathic practitioners to take the whole case, to understand the whole story, and to prescribe for the whole person. Our results tend to be more impressive and longer lasting when we aim broadly and prescribe accordingly.

New Year's Resolutions: Increasing Energy and Resolve

Our health is a product of our genetic inheritance, our lifestyle choices and the environment in which we live, work and play. Because we cannot alter our genetic inheritance (at least at this time), our best bets are to choose wisely in the way we live and to minimize our exposure to environmental toxins in our food, water and air. Other, less measurable toxins that are also best limited include negative thinking and unconstructive responses to stress.

We frequently see patients who stay in unsupportive relationships or unsatisfying jobs that may add to the maintaining causes of the pathology that brings them into the practitioner's office. Sometimes when I see a patient, I think, "This person doesn't just need a homeopathic remedy, they need a whole new living environment."

What can constitutional homeopathy offer when the thing that's really needed is a big change in health habits, relationships or livelihood? In my experience, the two things homeopathy can effectively offer are: clear resolve and an enhanced energy level.

During the season when New Year's resolutions abound, I am often audience to my patients' declarations about what they intend to do or not do, to begin or end, or to otherwise shift in the coming year. When patients return and report on the changes they were able to make as they felt better, had more energy, and gained needed confidence, I am overjoyed.

When they tell me about the healthy choices they made or a newfound ability to quell the torrents of negative thinking, I am the cheerleader on the sidelines.

I am reminded of a patient, who came to see me about fifteen years ago. Claire was thirty years old and single, an administrative assistant who struggled with seasonal allergies, premenstrual syndrome, excess weight and a nagging long term depression that kept her from enjoying her work, family and friends. She was treated successfully over several years with the homeopathic remedy *Natrum muriaticum* which matched both the way she experienced her allergies with lots of clear nasal discharge, much sneezing, and terribly chapped lips and her premenstrual syndrome with acne, sadness before the flow and being worse from consolation. *Natrum muriaticum* also nicely matched her overall character, her sensitive nature, and her conscientiousness at work and at home.

Claire was doing well overall and I did not see her for a number of years. She returned in crisis, however, with severe, chronic, debilitating sinusitis and recurrent styes. Her life had changed dramatically in the interceding years; she had married a man who had fallen gravely ill soon after their wedding. In his illness, he had become viciously faultfinding as well as verbally and emotionally abusive. (I would have loved to prescribe for him!) Claire had strong religious convictions and felt that divorce was not an option.

We worked together over several months to address the problems that seemed most limiting: her styes and sinusitis. We used homeopathic remedies as well as strong and effective naturopathic approaches such as hydrotherapy, botanical medicine and therapeutic nutrition. I was disappointed in our results; they were neither long lasting nor did they work preventively as they had with countless previous patients. I sent Claire for further diagnostic tests to be sure I was not missing other issues. The Eye-Ear-Nose-Throat specialist confirmed our diagnosis and reminded us that the allergic component was also a factor.

Alas, I came to realize that being and staying sick was Claire's way of manifesting her deep seated frustration with her life situation. The immense anger, resentment, sadness and disappointment at the core of her marriage provided an endless source of negative thoughts and bad feelings. I believe that Claire felt trapped and unable to make the needed changes—all part of why she was getting and staying sick. When I spoke to her directly about this idea, she at first resisted, then slowly recognized, and ultimately embraced this notion as a central truth to her unhappiness.

Claire would have to leave this man, and it would not be easy. The emotional, economic and domestic intertwining of their ten years together was complicated and profound; such a move went against her every moral fiber. This would be a slow and deliberate separation with much planning and forethought. She needed a supportive team of family and friends in addition to a well-prescribed homeopathic remedy to guide and support such a monumental shift in her self-definition, relationship status and living situation. As she began to draw plans for her new year as a single woman supporting herself, I looked for a remedy that could reduce her tendency for infections, lift her depressed spirits, and offer her the determination she would need to make the difficult changes ahead.

Claire needed tremendous attention and support over many months. We cannot provide this for all of our patients all of the time, yet most every homeopath has some patients for whom the healing relationship itself is another key to the mending of their life. Would Claire have improved without a homeopathic remedy? Would she have moved along as needed with only talk therapy? Perhaps. It seems to me, however, that by using her physical pathologies as a guide and seeing them in the context of her overall mental and emotional health, a specific and exact remedy was found that helped Claire in a more timely fashion. After all, she had been in this difficult living situation for years and had been working with a therapist, yet she'd still been unable to take those critical steps. How lucky we are to have a truly holistic medicine to offer our patients, and then to stand back and watch the results!

I gave Claire the remedy *Staphysagria* in ascending potencies to shore up her resolve and to help her build a stronger, healthier sense of self. This is a remedy well known for curing chronic and recurrent styes anywhere around the eyes. It is also known for helping the kind of headaches she got—a sense of fullness in the back of the head (occiput) that accompanied her sinusitis. Those headaches were always worse from anger or after an altercation with her husband; so even though the pathology was clearly physical, Claire's emotions were a part of it all—and a part of the *Staphysagria* symptom profile as well. She also had the keynote *Staphysagria* symptom of being worse after a nap.

After taking a dose of *Staphysagria,* Claire often commented that she felt it boosted her resolve, quieted what she called her 'negative-mind-talk,' and gave her the confidence to do the difficult things she had to do. Once Claire had made up her mind, she did not waver or look back. As she went through the process of making changes in her living situation and relationship, we both noticed that her sinusitis and styes became less and less of an issue. She had fewer infections, which were less severe and of shorter duration. As we often see with a well-prescribed homeopathic remedy, Claire's mental and emotional health improved; at the same time, she regained her energy, vision and resolve to make the necessary changes in her life.

At this time of year when I am privy to the New Year's aspirations of many a patient—sometimes around food or smoking, sometimes about the need to communicate better with a friend or partner, sometimes about beginning a realistic exercise program—I try to be encouraging and supportive. I express my preference for small incremental changes that can become permanent, and stress the fact our health (especially with regard to food, alcohol and exercise) reflects the habitual, not the occasional.

When huge life-altering changes are what is needed, as in Claire's case, I try to help troubleshoot and break the big projects into smaller more manageable pieces. I speak to the chance of new beginnings that the first of the year offers—and to the never-ending possibility for change, made doable by the resiliency of the human spirit. I always look for a broad reaching constitutional remedy that might help address the complaints at hand while simultaneously offering that dynamic combination: a bit more energy and a lot more resolve!

Stress and Pain: A Case of Costochondritis

I always tell my children, "It's not what you do with a good day, it's what you do with a bad one that matters." Stress is all around us: at home, in school, at work, in our communities and in our relationships. How we handle stress and what we do to minimize it are important factors in many of the illnesses homeopaths treat.

Where would we be without stress? Dead! Stressors keep us moving, keep us reconfiguring our lives, and keep us evolving as people and as a species. If there were no stressors, there would be no growth. We have come to understand stress as something negative, but as a more general term, it is everything in life to which we must react.

The daily stresses of living make some people more susceptible to the acute illnesses 'going around.' And the more intense stresses of demanding job situations, difficult relationships, and the world-at-large cause many to succumb to those problems for which they have some susceptibility, due to genetics and/or long term lifestyle factors. I wind up spending much of my time with patients talking about the stressors in their lives and helping them strategize how to reduce the amount and types of stress. At the same time, I try to help them figure out how to let off steam in order to counter the effects of stresses that cannot be avoided.

Understanding stress in the context of biology helps me as a homeopath. A patient's symptoms—physical, mental and emotional—are, in part, reactions to the stressors in their lives. Understanding the cycle of stress and the pathology it generates helps lead me to the correct remedy. I often tell my students that it is not about understanding the stress per se, but rather, how that stress specifically impacts the particular patient in question. It is essential that we not jump to conclusions based on our own experience of certain kinds of stress. For instance, if I have a patient who has recently lost a partner,

I need to ask about how that loss influenced them, instead of assuming any particular kind of response. In short, the nature of the stress itself is less important than the individualized response to it.

What follows is a brief case of a woman under tremendous job strain and how she handled it. This case illustrates how unrelenting stress in a susceptible person eventually takes its toll.

Shelia, a 45 year old lawyer at a high powered law firm where working 80 hours a week was common and expected, had forgone family and marriage and had poured her passion into her work instead. A few years back, she began to suffer from severe costochondritis—inflammation of the joint between the sternum and the clavicle and/or rib heads. Shelia felt like she was having repeated heart attacks, but after a thorough medical work-up, she was handed this diagnosis instead. She had constant sharp pain in a small area where the bones met. Sometimes it was worse with motion, sometimes worse being still. It was often worse in the middle of the night. It was a very intense pain that was not helped by over-the-counter anti-inflammatory medications. She had worked with chiropractors and physical therapists and had seen minimal improvement, but the severe pain and discomfort were getting the best of her. In addition, this situation precluded her participation in competitive athletics—a fine way she had historically countered her stressful lifestyle.

Shelia's job expectations along with the pain itself caused her tremendous anxiety, and the anxiety seemed to make the pain worse. She became worried about her own death—costochondritis is never life threatening—which led to terrible insomnia. The lack of sleep then became another trigger for the costochondritis. When she didn't sleep well, Shelia was aware, not surprisingly, that her law work suffered. This led her to work more hours, albeit less efficiently, which again led to more stress and a worsening of her overall condition, a cycle of pathology where things continued to worsen.

I set out to find a remedy that could address the type of pain Shelia had (localized and intense) along with the ensuing anxiety and insomnia. After taking her full case history including a review of systems, her physical general symptoms, and her family history, I prescribed *Kalium carbonicum* 200c, one dose. Besides the above-mentioned symptoms, I had learned that Shelia's pain was exacerbated in the middle of the night (*Kalium carbonicum* patients are often worse from 2:00–4:00 a.m.), and somewhat ameliorated if she sat up and leaned forward, another keynote of this remedy. The particular combination of intense, stitching pain and these modalities in a chilly person, one who craves sweets and experiences mounting anxiety, often leads me to this remedy choice.

I also recommended mild, natural anti-inflammatories: Bromelain, derived from pineapple, and Curcumin, derived from tumeric. I generally suggest 250 mg of each, three times a day, for musculoskeletal problems where inflammation is the main concern. Before prescribing I ask if the patient has any known allergy to either pineapple or tumeric and do not offer these adjunctive therapies if they do. I have not found these supplements to be miraculous, but they do seem to support the body's effort to reduce inflammation, without any of the side effects or potential damage to the liver associated with overuse of non-steroidal, anti-inflammatory medication.

These nutritional approaches do not, in my experience, antidote homeopathic medicines. They do not work as deeply as homeopathic remedies; rather, they take the edge off an intense inflammatory complaint. They will not impact the mental or emotional sphere of a patient and don't seem to enhance energy level or mental clarity. By contrast, what I would expect from the correct homeopathic remedy is that this patient would have fewer incidences and a lessening of the severity of the costochondritis, as well as less anxiety in general and better sleep. With that improved and consistent sleep, Shelia's energy and outlook should also improve. Moreover, I had a long conversation with her about the necessity of pulling back some from her work and finding non-stressful ways to relax and enjoy life.

When Shelia came to see me six weeks later, she reported that she'd had a handful of milder episodes but was feeling much better. Her sleep had improved dramatically because the pain wasn't waking her. Enhanced sleep goes a long way to supporting the healing process, and not surprisingly, her anxiety had also been greatly reduced. Shelia had begun to take a more serious look at the stressors in her life and to cut back at work.

Some six months later, during a time when Shelia was working against a difficult deadline, she had a flare-up of the costochondritis. We repeated the *Kalium carbonicum* 200c once, and two years on she is no longer plagued by costochondritis. Through her own efforts, her work with a counselor, and her constitutional homeopathic treatment, she has continued to recognize her early signs of too much stress. When she begins to experience such symptoms as mild insomnia and some indigestion, she acts on those observations by cutting back at work and doing some things that help her relax. Because she is pain-free, she is also able to participate in athletics again.

Stress isn't all bad—it's what we do with it and how we use it that counts!

Facing Cancer: What Can We Do?

In the mid-1990s, I had the pleasure of meeting Gene, a 60 year old, retired postal worker, who came to me for a consultation. Eleven months earlier, this gentle, kind man had been diagnosed with pancreatic cancer with metastasis to the liver and with lymphocytic leukemia. This was not good news for anyone. The fact that Gene was one month from retirement at the time of diagnosis was heartbreaking. He and his wife had been through a lot over the years and had been looking forward to this time of life.

Surgeons had removed a primary tumor in Gene's abdomen, and he was taking medication to try to slow the growth of the cancer, but his oncologists had told him a cure could not be expected at this late stage in his illness. Gene was now experiencing abdominal pain that radiated to his back. It felt like heartburn, and burping helped some. The pain was worse when he sat up and worse the more he thought about it. For years, Gene had had terrific pains across the front of his abdomen that were worse from eating peanuts, potato chips, or other high fat foods, and occasionally, he would still have those pains.

Gene had come to me for help in relieving his digestive pains, improving his comfort, and enjoying his life for as long as he could. I went to work taking his homeopathic case, listening to his story, and trying to understand the symptoms as he described them—how they fit into his health history and how they fit into his overall life at the time of our visit. Gene's wife was very helpful, offering information along the way and lovingly supporting her husband of nearly forty years.

I don't know whether this is true for other homeopaths, but during my earlier years of practice, I saw many pregnant women, young children and growing families. I still see such folks, but as my patient population has aged, I seem to be seeing more patients with serious pathology, including cancer. What is the role of the homeopath when a patient comes to us with a cancer diagnosis? What can we expect homeopathy and other natural medicines to do for such a patient?

In my experience, homeopathic and other natural medicine care is extremely helpful, whether used at the time of diagnosis, during conventional cancer treatment or afterward for healing and prevention of further disease. That said, I believe that, in general, an integrative approach is best. No one practitioner has all the answers. No one healing philosophy has to be embraced to the exclusion of others. And thankfully, there is now increased availability and access to information on how to take the best from seemingly different healing paradigms. What is most important is to be sure there is full disclosure on all sides, so all practitioners and physicians understand what treatment approaches the patient is using.

We homeopaths treat each patient individually. With cancer, as with any illness, we have no set homeopathic remedies to give based on say, what type of cancer the person has or where the cancer is. There is no list to go check against and prescribe accordingly. Oh how we sometimes wish there were! But homeopathy's beauty, its challenge, and ultimately its promise, is to find medicines that fit the particular patient at a particular point in time.

To the newer homeopathic prescribers that I train, a patient with cancer can seem daunting. The stakes seem higher, but in truth, we use the very same tools of the trade; it is careful case taking and the understanding of all aspects of the patient that will lead to the best remedy possible.

Patients recently diagnosed with cancer usually come to me looking for help and information to get through surgery, chemotherapy and radiation, and to deal with the emotional impact of a cancer diagnosis. They are hoping to reduce side effects and increase the efficacy of the conventional medical approaches they are using.

Many other patients come to see me a year or two after their conventional cancer treatments have been completed. These patients usually fall into one of two categories:

1. Those who report that even though they have survived cancer and the treatments, they just do not feel well (perhaps they are tired, or feel they are not thinking clearly, or maybe they aren't sleeping well or feel depressed) and
2. Those who feel well enough but are seeking all the help they can find to prevent recurrence of the cancer.

Still other patients, like Gene, arrive at my office in more advanced stages of illness with strong symptoms from the cancer itself—perhaps in the digestive tract or the respiratory tract or the musculoskeletal system. They are seeking symptom relief and an improved quality of life for as long as possible.

Each of these patients is unique and each must be addressed individually. Sometimes their prognosis is very good and sometimes it is dire, but I find that there is almost always some help that we can offer.

In my experience, an integrative approach to treating cancer is best. For those wanting to receive such treatment under one roof, I have referred numerous patients to The Cancer Treatment Centers of America (CTCA). Their website notes that CTCA: 'combines the latest medical, surgical and radiological therapies with supportive therapies like nutrition, mind-body medicine, physical therapy, naturopathy and spiritual wellness, bringing to bear many novel and innovative weapons against your specific type of cancer.' CTCA has hospitals or treatment facilities in Zion, Illinois, Philadelphia, Pennsylvania, Tulsa, Oklahoma and Seattle, Washington, and nearby Phoenix, Arizona. For further information see their website at www.cancercenter.com.

Many patients who are diagnosed with cancer are seemingly asymptomatic. For example, a breast lump might have been discovered on a mammogram, or a prostate cancer may have been diagnosed after a blood test showed elevated PSA (prostate-specific antigen). For these patients, who have typically undergone surgery or other treatment before seeing me, I generally take the full homeopathic case and prescribe a constitutional remedy; I will include my understanding of the cancer in my analysis, but I am also intent on understanding it in the context of the patient's overall health, how their various bodily systems are functioning (for example, digestion, circulation, etc.), and their physical general symptoms. (Alicia, described later, is an example of such a patient.)

The stress of receiving a cancer diagnosis itself is often enough to push a patient toward a lower level of health. So, for example, a patient who tended toward allergies and eczema when under stress might experience these symptoms to a greater degree than ever before. We might say that the stress has pushed the person deeper into their constitutional remedy state; and they would benefit from a dose of whatever constitutional remedy they needed before the cancer diagnosis.

Sometimes, however, the stress of the diagnosis is so great or it perhaps triggers such an intense response due to family or personal history, that the patient is bumped into another state of health altogether. That is, instead of (or in addition to) a worsening of their usual symptoms of allergies and eczema, they might develop new and more troublesome symptoms like heart and circulatory problems. In such a case, this person would probably benefit from a different constitutional remedy than the one they might have needed before their cancer diagnosis.

Typically, however, I do not have the certainty of knowing what constitutional remedy the person needed prior to diagnosis because most who come to me with cancer are new patients. (Like many practicing homeopaths, I find that the rate of cancer among the patients that I have been treating for many years is rather low.)

Then there are the patients who come to me with strong symptoms from the cancer, perhaps based on where the cancer is located in the body, or symptoms that arise during conventional treatment. This person might also benefit from their constitutional remedy if the current symptoms are within the purview of that remedy. For instance, perhaps I have a patient who has done well over the years with the remedy *Phosphorus* on a constitutional level and is now undergoing chemotherapy for breast cancer. She may develop more symptoms, such as easy bruising and extreme fatigue due to her treatments, but she still remains open in her demeanor, in need of affection and attention, and very thirsty. She may be more intensely anxious and be struggling with diarrhea, a new symptom for her. But since each of her issues is still well covered by the remedy *Phosphorus*, I would give her *Phosphorus* again.

We can view the receipt of a cancer diagnosis, the cancer itself, and conventional cancer treatments each as stressors on the system. Most people respond to stressors in predictable and patterned ways, as in the previous example of the woman who would benefit from another dose of her constitutional remedy, *Phosphorus*. But those who respond by developing new symptoms not covered by their usual or former constitutional remedy will need a different prescription. If, for example, this same woman develops easy bruising and bothersome diarrhea, but she also becomes extra anxious, critical, and difficult to please, this represents a shift in her predictable pattern of response.

Her new symptoms may signal that instead of *Phosphorus*, she now needs *Arsenicum album* since the new symptoms are more in line with the indications for this remedy.

Nonetheless, I do not have preconceived ideas about how I will prescribe, except that I will look for the most broadly acting remedy to support the patient in the broadest possible way. I will be alert to the possibility that another remedy may be indicated, especially during the course of conventional treatment, based on how the patient responds to those approaches.

It is fine to have patients use homeopathic medicines right alongside their conventional cancer treatments. I often use a low strength remedy such as a 12c potency, repeated once or twice a day, although I sometimes use a higher potency, such as one dose of 200c, if I think the patient might not remember to take a daily dose. I generally follow up with patients getting conventional treatments more frequently; the worse they feel, the sooner I want to hear back from them or see them again. I instruct them to call me if side effects from conventional treatment are becoming intolerable, if their spirits are really taking a hit, or if other seemingly acute illnesses arise during conventional treatment.

Gene had lost 36 pounds after his surgery but had put back on 20 during his recuperation. Since the tumor, Gene reported sweating profusely on his back and head at night in bed and needing to have a fan blow on him continuously. His labored breathing was obvious in the office that day. He had difficulty climbing stairs, felt short of breath, and felt weak especially through the knees, arms, shoulders and hips. He would get bad cramps in his legs and in his hands, which were worse since he'd been placed on prednisone.

His spleen was enlarged, and he had fainted several times in the last few months. When he was younger, he would pass out at the sight of blood. He had terrible gas ever since the surgery, with constant belching and passing gas, which offered some relief. He had bowel movements two or three times a day, and he desired sweet and salty foods. He had a poor sense of smell and taste and was not especially thirsty.

Gene had a history of smoking a pack of cigarettes a day, but he'd stopped some 20 years ago. He had never been a big drinker of alcohol. He'd had thyroid cancer in his forties. He had high blood pressure.

When asked to describe his temperament he said, 'I am a pussycat. It takes a lot to get me going. I don't need friends too much, although I have a few and enjoy them.' Gene was very pleasant throughout our conversation, supporting his wife at every turn, holding her hand, and being incredibly upbeat considering his grave diagnosis and prognosis.

The severe nature of Gene's shortness of breath with his need for constant fanning, coupled with his increasing digestive distress with a lot of gas that was somewhat relieved by belching, would point most experienced homeopaths to the remedy *Carbo vegetabilis,* since these are strong indications for this remedy. Overall weakness and debility is also something we see in patients who need *Carbo vegetabilis,* along with a tendency towards fainting.

Gene received much help from this remedy within the week. He gained immediate strength and was even able to resume his model airplane hobby. He was better able to breathe and his problem with gas was greatly reduced; he still had flatulence, but it was limited to the after-dinner hour and it was not as intense or long lasting. I told him to call if other problems arose.

Had he needed *Carbo vegetabilis* years earlier, before he developed cancer? His history of digestive symptoms and easy fainting could point to that. Or perhaps he had needed *Lycopodium* earlier (a remedy often used constitutionally for those with chronic digestive issues), and his illness had pushed him into a *Carbo vegetabilis* state. It is hard to know for certain, as I had never treated him before.

Gene next came to see me two months later when he reported that although he'd done well for most of the time since our last visit, he was now in a lot of pain. There did not seem to be any position, activity or medication that would relieve him, and he felt like he could not bear it any longer. He described incessant, strong gas pains; added to that, he was unable to get a good breath. And he had begun to receive further chemotherapy. I believed that he had experienced a relapse along with a continuation of his progressive pathology, so I gave *Carbo vegetabilis* in a higher strength. Within days of taking the remedy, he reported that the pain was under control and his breathing improved.

The homeopathic remedies continued to give Gene symptomatic relief over the course of six months and reduced his need for opiate painkillers with their unwanted effects, for which he and his family were grateful. Gene did die of his cancer, and I treated him right up and through that time with more *Carbo vegetabilis*, and then with *Arsenicum album*, when his anxiety, fear of death and restlessness were more than he could bear. After each dose of the *Arsenicum*, his wife would report that Gene seemed more comfortable, less agitated and clearer mentally. She was very thankful for our work together, as it gave her husband some peace at the end. This pattern of needing one remedy, then perhaps another, and then winding up at *Arsenicum album* as a person nears death, though not universal, is certainly common. While it is not easy to experience the death of a patient, it is comforting to have helped to make his last days as calm as possible.

Alicia, another patient who came to see me in the 1990s, was diagnosed earlier in the disease process than Gene had been, and her story has had a happier ending. At age 45, she was just hitting her stride as a lawyer and active mother of two robust teenage sons when she found a cancerous lump in her left breast. She had a lumpectomy (no metastasis was detected) followed by chemotherapy and 28 radiation treatments. She came to see me a half-year later, while putting together what she called her 'dream team' of advisors, doctors, therapists, family and friends.

Alicia had taken on her diagnosis and treatment plan with energy and organization. At the time of our first visit, her main request was that I help her to 'keep healthy so the cancer won't come back.' She also wanted relief from the swelling (lymphedema) in her arm on the same side where she had had the surgery and radiation. She told me that since her treatments, she'd been suffering with a full body rash that was red, slightly raised and itchy, and worse when she became warm, especially after a shower, while in bed or if she was out walking.

Alicia's health history was remarkably good. She was a long time vegetarian, who had been running and doing yoga regularly for decades. She had no family history of cancer, and most of her relatives lived into their eighties and nineties. The irony of her diagnosis did not seem to bother her. 'Look, bad things happen to good people,' she told me, and she was just going to 'get on with it' and do what she could to live a healthy and long life.

I took Alicia's homeopathic case and prescribed the remedy *Sulphur*. My reasons included these classic *Sulphur* indications:

the left sidedness of her complaint; an itchy bothersome skin rash that was worse from heat; her outgoing and upbeat nature; and the fact that, aside from the breast cancer, she was quite healthy.

I also instructed her on how to alternate hot and cold soaks to her left hand to get the circulation going along with the physical therapy she was already getting. In addition, I created a vitamin-mineral-botanical medicine program based on her history, her diet, and her willingness to make certain lifestyle changes.

A month later, Alicia returned to my office to say that the swelling and range of motion were improving steadily on her left side and that she was feeling good. The rash, while still visible, was fading and no longer itchy. Alicia was pleased with these results, and I judged that the *Sulphur* was acting well.

For the past ten years, I have worked with Alicia on and off through the changes of her chemotherapy-induced menopause, acute infections, allergies, and the launching of her children out of the nest. Sometimes I prescribe a homeopathic remedy. *Sulphur* has continued to be a very helpful remedy for her, when indicated, sometimes other naturopathic treatments.

Alicia has remained free of the cancer and has learned much about taking care of herself. In the process I have learned much, too: to step forward and treat patients who have or have had cancer by using the same tools I use with all my patients, but at the same time to keep up with the current research on cancer and its treatments—and to try to do it all with confidence and grace.

Between early diagnoses, aggressive allopathic approaches, and our complementary and alternative medicine offerings, many people with cancer live long and healthy, productive lives, post-diagnosis. In my 22 years of experience, I have found homeopathic care to be very beneficial for patients with cancer—used at the time of diagnosis, during conventional treatment, and afterward for healing and prevention of further disease.

Ménière's: A Dizzying Disease

When Polly first came into my office in the late 1990s, she was short on stature but long on intensity. A former competitive skater, she had the trim body and keen passion of an elite athlete. As a mother, homemaker, and human resource manager, Polly kept a full and busy schedule, so a diagnosis of Ménière's disease a year before our initial visit was severely impacting her life.

Her chief complaint was severe dizziness that would not allow her to get out of bed for days at a time; she simply could not move without total loss of balance, severe nausea, and vomiting. Add to that the terrible ringing in her ears and moderate hearing loss, and Polly was feeling far from her fit and active self.

By the time I saw Polly, the bouts were getting closer together, from every three to four months to every three to four weeks. For this woman who had thought nothing of whirling and spinning in tighter and tighter circles on the thin blade of a skate, the inability to get out of bed, make her daughter breakfast, and tend to other daily duties was totally unacceptable.

Named after a nineteenth century French physician, Ménière's disease is a disorder of the inner ear that affects both the areas of balance (vestibular labyrinth) and hearing (cochlea). Most people with the illness experience periodic episodes of extreme dizziness, along with tinnitus (ringing, buzzing, roaring in the ear) and hearing loss. Over time, patients may have fewer problems with balance but may be left with residual hearing loss and bothersome tinnitus. Usually, only one ear is affected, but that is little consolation to the sufferer. Approximately 100,000 new cases of Ménière's are diagnosed each year in the United States.

Although the causes of this illness are unknown, many theories have been advanced. An increase in fluid pressure in the inner ear is believed to be involved; perhaps there is a degradation of cochlear or vestibular hair cells due to shifts in production and absorption of the fluid (endolymph) that bathes the inner ear. Conditions that cause narrowing of blood vessels to the area may also be implicated. Cases of Ménière's have been reported after injury to the head or bouts of middle ear infection. Many women suffering with Ménière's have noticed that attacks are more likely in the week leading up to the menstrual flow. A genetic predisposition may also be a factor.

Diagnosis of Ménière's disease is based on the patient's clinical presentation. Audiometric studies can test hearing, and a myriad of other diagnostic tools, such as CT scan and MRI, can confirm the diagnosis. A number of other disorders must be ruled out, such as acoustic neuroma or tumor (which can produce the same symptoms), labyrinthitis (dizziness due to inflammation of the labyrinth, usually resolving on its own in four to six weeks and not accompanied by tinnitus and hearing loss), hypertension, carotid artery disease, multiple sclerosis, anemia, and others.

Conventional medicine views Ménière's as a progressive illness that is essentially incurable; conventional treatment focuses on symptom relief through drug therapy, vestibular rehabilitation therapy, and as a last resort, surgery. Medications recommended for long term treatment include diuretics to decrease fluids in the body, antihistamines, and sedatives. Salt restriction is usually advised, less than two grams per day. For those who suffer over time with unrelenting and incapacitating vertigo, surgery in which the labyrinth on the affected side is permanently destroyed does relieve symptoms, but comes with a hefty price tag: total and irreversible hearing loss.

As with most any chronic disease, no two patients experience their Ménière's in exactly the same way. Whenever I take a case history and see the individual stamp that a patient puts on their pathology, I feel blessed to be a homeopath. I know that I can take these unique, individualizing bits of information and actually use them to determine an effective remedy. In order to gather this information, I ask my Ménière's patients the following kinds of questions:

- When did the Ménière's begin? Was there a clear etiology, cause or starting point?
- Can you describe how you feel during an attack?
- Is there something that tends to bring on an attack?
- Is there anything you can do during an attack to gain relief?
- Are there other, seemingly unrelated symptoms that arise during an attack?

- Can you describe how the noises in the ear sound?
- Is the hearing loss worse for certain sounds?
- Are there times when the hearing loss seems worse?

Finally, I always ask the patient: What is the worst thing about having this problem? I ask all my patients with chronic illness this question, and it often surprises them. Why do I ask it? Because sometimes as we are hearing a recounting of a patient's story, we project onto their situation our own feelings, ideas, or beliefs about what we think would be the worst part of having this illness; but the patient may have a totally different perspective.

For example, one of my Ménière's patients answered this question in a way that I would never have anticipated. 'I'm embarrassed. When my balance is off, I fear that people will think I'm drunk,' she replied. 'My father was an alcoholic and this brings up a tremendous amount of shame for me.' This was an important piece of information to help me understand this patient and how the Ménière's was playing out in her life, and it ultimately helped to point me toward a curative remedy for her.

In addition to the above questions, I always do a complete review of bodily systems (for example digestive, musculoskeletal, etc.), making sure to understand the patient's physical general symptoms: food cravings and aversions, thirst, body temperature, weather preferences, time of day of aggravations or exacerbations and sleep position. I also ask about mental and emotional tendencies, fears, anxieties, ability to do their work, etc.

Although Polly had come to see me based on a friend's strong recommendation, she didn't shy away from saying that it was also a last resort. She was what I affectionately call, 'skeptical but desperate.' She had an analytical mind and was deeply entrenched in the world of conventional medicine, as her father was a physician. Until now, however, she had enjoyed good health and a strong vitality, and in general, had had little need for the medical world.

Polly brought a year's worth of notes on her illness neatly typed and duplicated so we could each have a copy in front of us as she reviewed her experiences and treatment attempts. She was dressed professionally, had a sensible haircut, and spoke articulately and with precision.

Polly reported that she'd taken the medications her doctors prescribed including a diuretic, an anti-vertigo medicine and an anti-nausea drug, all to no avail. With this illness, her life had become severely restricted in almost every way. Her energy was flagging; tasks that required exertion were beyond her. Her thinking was not as clear, and perhaps most disturbing to her, everything at home and at work was falling apart. Things were a mess, with piles everywhere, deadlines zipping by and projects uncompleted.

Polly's first episode of Ménière's had begun the previous year after a very stressful time at work. She had had an intense upper respiratory tract infection that had lasted for about two months. She had taken antibiotics and 'crawled' her way back to health. A few weeks later, she had started feeling somewhat dizzy, and it got progressively worse. When she had the vertigo, she had to lie perfectly still with her eyes closed. If she did not want to vomit, she could not turn her head or move her eyes at all. She had a persistent hum in her left ear that was very distracting. That ear also had a reduced level of hearing, which she mostly noticed while talking on the phone.

Polly's anxiety about her health, which she had a healthy dose of anyway, was heightened. She worried a lot. What if she had a brain tumor? What if she died, what would happen to her daughter? In the past, if she were feeling anxious, she would get up and do something: exert herself, tidy up, or just go for a walk. But with the Ménière's, these stress reducers were not an option. She seemed to be worsening as the months went by, and she felt out of control and on the verge of anxiety all the time.

In general, Polly was chilly, would sweat easily on exertion, and tended to be constipated. Her husband described her as a neat freak and a bit of a control freak. Polly disagreed, stating that she just liked things to be in order. It helped her to be more efficient and productive if things were in place in her home, her office, her car, and when she had a neatly printed schedule of the day's events along with her 'to-do' list.

I appreciated Polly's earnestness, her directness and her ability to describe her pathology so carefully. Many of her symptoms as well as much of her overall temperament and her physical characteristics are easily found in the repertory. This book, which indexes almost all the symptoms known to humanity and the homeopathic remedies known to help them, is rich in information for the homeopath, especially with regard to Ménière's. The Vertigo section is short but filled with all the symptoms and modalities one could imagine about dizziness. In fact, for those unfamiliar with this illness, a ramble through the repertory gives a scenic tour of the myriad unpleasant possibilities that may plague someone with Ménière's.

When I look back through my files at the last five patients

who came in with the chief complaint of Ménière's disease, I find that each received a different remedy: *Nux moschata, Calcarea carbonica, Staphysagria, Argentum nitricum,* and *Conium maculatum.* This illustrates the point that, for those suffering with Ménière's, as with most chronic diseases, the homeopathic remedy that will offer relief and gradual but permanent improvement will not be chosen in a 'cookbook' fashion. I need to take the full case in order to understand all the minutiae of the way the patient experiences their vertigo, ear noises and hearing loss. I then need to step back and view all that in the context of the person's overall health. In so doing, I am privy to the promise of homeopathy: tailoring medicines to individual people who have individual sicknesses. How challenging and gratifying for the homeopath! And when the prescription is successful, how helpful for the patient!

Based on the qualities of Polly's vertigo (inability to move without nausea and dizziness, worse moving her eyes), her physical general symptoms (constipation, chilliness), and her temperament (ultra-organized, controlling), I prescribed *Calcarea carbonica* 200c, one pellet, one time. As a naturopathic physician, I was also happy to offer her other natural medicine approaches listed below.

Polly came to see me some four weeks later. She was elated as she'd not had an episode since taking the *Calcarea carbonica.* I was happy for her, too, but not quite as enthusiastic, since I knew she might have had four good weeks regardless of treatment. I prescribed no homeopathic remedy but advised her to continue taking the natural supplements, return to see me in another six weeks, and call if she had another episode.

Six weeks went by and, at her follow-up visit, Polly

reported that she'd felt like she was going to have an attack the previous week—but it had never materialized. She said that she'd had an easier menstrual cycle with less PMS and wondered if that could have been because of the homeopathic treatment and the supplements she was taking. This sort of positive shift in health occurring in an area that the patient had not sought care for is a common occurrence after a well-prescribed homeopathic remedy. Perhaps the B vitamins and magnesium were also helping in this regard.

Over the last seven years, Polly has occasionally come to see me for acute illnesses and once for a mild recurrence of the vertigo symptoms, but by and large she has remained well after several doses of *Calcarea carbonica* spread out over the seven years and prescribed as needed. Polly would come in on occasion and say, 'Okay doc, I need a tune up.' What she meant was that she did not feel as well, her energy was going down, or perhaps her Ménière's symptoms were starting to creep back. Another dose of *Calcarea carbonica* would set her back on track. In all, she had three doses of *Calcarea carbonica* 200c and two doses of *Calcarea carbonica* 1M over those seven years. She never again had a severe bout with the dizziness. In addition, and to the amazement of her eye-ear-nose-throat doctor, Polly's hearing returned to normal and the ringing in her ears also stopped.

Like many a former skeptic, Polly has become one of the most zealous supporters of homeopathy and often sends me friends and relatives to treat. Of course, not all of them experience the fast and complete resolution of their problems as Polly did. Her good results are likely because she had a strong constitution that manifested an illness with clarity and strength. When a patient produces such clear symptoms, it is typically easier for a homeopath to find the correct remedy, and the prognosis for the patient is also very good. Over the years, however, I have found that most of my patients with Ménière's do very well. With homeopathic treatment, they report fewer or no further episodes of dizziness, great reduction or disappearance of ringing in the ears, as well as a complete or partial return to normal hearing.

One day recently, when the pond in our neighborhood had finally frozen over, I had the great pleasure of watching Polly out on the ice. She had the powerful grace of a heron in flight, arms outstretched, and the wide smile on her face catching the sun. As I gingerly made my way across the ice, Polly glided gracefully toward me and executed one of those sharp, skidding stops. She gave me a short (unsuccessful) lesson in skating backwards, and then she was off like a flash. I was left to contemplate the power of homeopathy and the sheer impact a simple, but elegant remedy can have, when prescribed with just the right touch.

Ménière's is a chronic disease, which will respond best to constitutional homeopathic care. That said, a few remedies do stand out as commonly prescribed ones:

Cocculus. The patient feels as if the room is spinning. They cannot get out of bed. They will be aggravated by being in any moving vehicle or even by watching something else move. They are often worse if they have lost sleep from whatever cause.

Phosphorus. The patient is worse first thing in the morning; worse sitting in a warm room. They are better lying on the right side and when they are able to get a good night's sleep.

They may develop Ménière's after loss of fluid from bleeding.

Conium maculatum. The patient is worse from turning over in bed and much better if they can lie still with their eyes shut. They are worse from sudden motion and better if they are left alone to rest.

Calcarea carbonica. The patient is worse from exertion of any kind; they may develop the condition from overwork and not enough sleep. Vertigo comes on when in high places or when looking up at others standing in a high place.

Argentum nitricum. Vertigo with a funny feeling in the head. Light-headedness and need for company. Unsteady gait. The patient feels like they are spinning even when sitting still.

More Natural Options

We can complement the work of homeopathic remedies with other gentle and effective treatments. Some patients choose to use only homeopathy, but for those with Ménière's who are interested in other natural medicine approaches, I recommend the following:

1. Vitamin C: 1000 mg, twice a day.
2. Bioflavonoids: 500 mg, twice a day.
3. Reduce salt intake to less than two grams a day.
4. B-complex vitamin: 50–100 mg per day.
5. Ginkgo biloba: Some studies have shown that taking this herb, 40 mg three times a day, will help with tinnitus.
6. Magnesium: 500 mg/day.

In general, my patients and I have been pleased with the natural medicine approaches in the care of Ménière's.

When Muscles, Bones and Joints Go Out of Whack

I recently viewed the IMAX movie *Wired to Win: Surviving the Tour de France*, an incredible feat of filmmaking that brings the human body into larger-than-life focus as it explores the interwoven anatomical and physiological precision required of riders in this demanding bicycle race. Using live-action footage and computerized medical imagery, the film examines concepts like endurance, graphically demonstrating how each person's brain responds to challenges.

Although I had the good fortune to study anatomy and physiology in depth in medical school (including lab work on a cadaver), I found this film to be an eye-opener. It brought to life the mechanical and chemical miracles at play in even the 'average' human in a most amazing way—how we take for granted when everything is working smoothly and how crazy making it can be when things break down.

Patients come to see me for many reasons, but as my clientele ages, I see more and more people with orthopedic complaints. The natural process of aging surely accounts for some of these problems, but others are the result of all the exercising baby-boomers are doing—in attempts to side-step that very aging process!

Many people come to me because they're not getting the results they seek from over the counter or prescription drugs, or because the drugs are causing intolerable side effects. Others worry that the medications may be addressing their pain, but that underlying joint degeneration and chronic inflammation are not being considered. More recently, patients seek alternatives in light of frightening news about some non-steroidal anti-inflammatory drugs. 'Can homeopathy offer me anything?' they ask. After twenty years of practice, I am happy to answer yes, and to share some thoughts with you about the homeopathic treatment of orthopedic complaints.

Like many classical homeopaths, I have treated a wide range of musculoskeletal complaints including: arthritis of the hands, wrists, shoulders, hips and knees, costochondritis, bunions, plantar fasciitis, stiff neck, carpal tunnel syndrome, back pain, and garden variety sports injuries like dislocating shoulders, sprained ankles, muscle cramps, shin splints and overuse syndromes. I also see patients who have orthopedic issues as part and parcel of more serious systemic disorders such as rheumatoid arthritis and lupus.

How do I treat patients with orthopedic problems? In just the same way that I treat patients with other kinds of complaints! I always look at the presenting issues in the context of the whole person. Not everyone with a sprained ankle needs *Arnica* and not everyone with back pain needs *Rhus toxicodendron*. The beauty of homeopathy is that we can individualize the treatment to the person, thereby getting better results.

Many turn away from homeopathy when it fails them, and it often fails them because they've chosen remedies in a cookbook fashion, based on scant few symptoms and not on the totality of the person with the complaint. Harder to prescribe this way? Possibly. More difficult to teach this approach? Certainly. More consistently effective? Absolutely!

So, if you have the opportunity to help someone with what seems like a simple, straight-forward musculoskeletal issue, don't shy away. Just remember: It is a complaint like any other, and it needs to be seen in the context of the whole patient. You need to do a simple review of systems (e.g., digestion, sleep, skin, mental/emotional sphere, etc.) to see if anything else has changed since the injury or illness. In this way, you are offering the best possible homeopathic care that lives up to the promise and elegance of homeopathy and takes the whole person into consideration.

Patients with orthopedic complaints often appear to be suffering from an acute problem, so our first job is to decide whether the complaint is truly acute or whether it's a manifestation of more chronic illness. If the patient has benefited from a particular constitutional remedy in the past, if the new symptoms are known to be helped by that remedy (based on remedy provings/clinical indications), and if the patient's physical general symptoms (for example body temperature, food cravings and aversions, thirst, sleep position, temperament, etc.) have not changed—then the person most likely needs a dose of their constitutional remedy. This can be true even if they have never had this complaint before.

For instance, I treat Annette, a lovely woman in her 70s, who has done well over the past decade with the constitutional remedy *Lycopodium* for the treatment of anxiety, irritability and irritable bowel syndrome (IBS). Some years into our work together, Annette began to complain of arthritic hands, and pain and stiffness in her wrists. Her IBS and her moods were now much improved, but this new symptom had arisen. I did a review of systems and of her physical general symptoms: Annette appeared to be the same as ever—still chilly, still preferring to sleep on her right side, still craving sweets, and still irritable if hungry or contradicted. She had no additional new symptoms.

I gave Annette another dose of *Lycopodium* to address her hand and wrist problems. It reduced the swelling and inflammation and enabled her to pick up where she had left off with several knitting and quilting projects—and to avoid using over-the-counter pain medicines. Just because Annette's hand and wrist symptoms were new, it did not necessarily mean that she needed a new remedy.

Another patient, 40 year old Renee came to see me for the first time complaining of plantar fasciitis, an incapacitating pain in the bottom of her left heel that made walking difficult and exercise impossible. This was wreaking havoc with her active lifestyle, her work as a nurse, and her ability to run her household with three school aged children. Upon taking her full case, I learned that Renee had other problems with inflammation, such as inflamed cold sores and sinus infections each winter. A sensitive and hard-working woman, loyal and caring to her husband and long-time friends, Renee also suffered from premenstrual migraines that sent her looking for her dark, quiet bedroom. These symptoms were consistent with indications for the homeopathic remedy *Natrum muriaticum.*

When I prescribed one dose of *Natrum muriaticum* 200c to treat Annette's fasciitis, the medical student sitting in with me that day asked why I had not chosen a remedy more specific to foot pain, as that was what was most limiting to Renee. I told him that I always prefer to give a broader, more holistically prescribed remedy if I can find one. Had this prescription not worked, I would have turned to remedies with a smaller sphere of influence that specifically address this type of pain, like *Ruta* or *Rhus toxicodendron*. Happily, over the course of a few months and with one more dose of *Natrum muriaticum* 200c, Renee's plantar fasciitis resolved—as did her migraine headaches. She has also had fewer sinus infections over the past several years.

Sometimes patients have true acute orthopedic problems that call for an acute homeopathic remedy. Jerry, a 45 year old pianist, had been my patient off and on for more than a decade. I had successfully treated him for chronic prostatitis, hay fever and skin problems with *Staphysagria* and more recently with *Pulsatilla*. He came to see me one day, bent over, unable to walk upright because of pain in his back. Out working in the garden the previous day, Jerry had noted nothing unusual—but the next morning he awakened unable to straighten up. He felt worse when he tried to move or take a deep breath.

I noticed that Jerry was decidedly curt with my receptionist and seemed impatient with me —a dramatic shift from his more easy going (that is, *Pulsatilla*) self. He also had changed from his generally thirstless nature to drinking incessantly throughout our interview. Because of this, I knew immediately that he had shifted from needing his constitutional remedy to needing a different, acute remedy, even though *Pulsatilla* certainly can be considered in treating backaches.

Once I determined that Jerry's lung sounds were normal, I gave him a dose of *Bryonia* 200c, a common acute remedy for back pain, when the pain is worse with motion, especially in a person who is irritable and dry, for example, dry lips, constipated and thirsty, all of which described Jerry to a T. Jerry called the next day to say he was much improved. Two days later, he was entirely back to normal. It is by locating the problem within the context of the individual that we are better able to prescribe accurately and with confidence. Jerry did revert back to his *Pulsatilla* state, a remedy I did not repeat routinely at that time, but rather some months later, when some of his more chronic issues began to resurface.

Over the years, I've noticed that people who need certain constitutional remedies tend to develop acute illnesses that respond to related remedies. For example, *Calcarea carbonica* types may develop acute problems that respond to *Rhus toxicodendron. Natrum muriaticum* constitutional types tend to develop acute problems that respond to *Bryonia*. Many other such relationships between remedies are noted in the homeopathic literature. If a person is given a dose of their indicated constitutional remedy, however, it can actually help shift them away from the tendency to get these acute problems in the first place.

For example, I often see people who have been self-treating their musculoskeletal problem with *Rhus toxicodendron* or *Bryonia* for years. Their sciatica or bursitis flares up periodically, they take their acute remedy, and the pain and inflammation go away in short order. They swear by their homeopathic acute remedy and wouldn't be without it. When they come to see me for treatment of a different complaint (for example constipation or sinusitis) and I give them their constitutional remedy, they are surprised to find their sciatica or bursitis attacks occurring much less frequently or disappearing altogether. By my aiming at a deeper level and prescribing a widely acting, constitutional remedy vs. an acute, more narrowly focused remedy, these patients get long-term relief.

Here's one last vignette. I was in a deep sleep one night many years ago, and my three, then small children were tucked in and dreaming. My husband was out of town, teaching overseas. In the wee hours of the morning, I was awakened by the distinctive sound of my front door creaking open. Heart throbbing, I grabbed my robe and a baseball bat as I headed downstairs to defend my offspring. 'Amy?' I heard a voice say. 'It's me, John.' A dear friend had let himself in, carrying his eight year old son who was having trouble breathing. I put down the baseball bat and asked what was going on. 'I know we should have gone to the emergency room,' explained John, 'but Robbie didn't want to go, he wanted to see if you could help first.' Great, I was thinking, the kid can barely breathe, it's three in the morning, and here we are in my living room, all of us bleary eyed. I ran for my stethoscope and, hearing good lung sounds, I happened to feel Robbie's spine as I was listening. Seemed a thoracic rib was way out of alignment. I asked Robbie to lie on the rug and did a simple adjustment to his back. Robbie sat up, took a deep breath, and said, 'Oh, that's much better!' He was asleep in his father's arms before they reached their car.

The moral of the story: A mechanical problem often needs a mechanical solution! It would be hard to imagine that even the perfectly prescribed homeopathic remedy would have relieved Robbie in this way.

That sort of story aside, with orthopedic issues, homeopathy can be applied just as it is applied in all cases—prescribed for the suffering individual, based on how the symptoms fit into the overall context of the patient. Determine if the problem is acute or chronic in nature; if it's the latter, remember that the constitutional remedy often will be just what the doctor ordered. And see if you can find that IMAX movie, you won't be disappointed!

Irregular Pap Tests, Genital Warts and Herpes

When I first saw Sherri's intake form, I was struck by how neatly and completely she had filled it out and described her chief complaint: 'I have genital warts, which have caused my Pap smears to be abnormal. I have needed to have biopsies to the area and a procedure to remove the top layers of my cervix. I also have herpes simplex in my genital area and suffer from monthly outbreaks. I have some history of mild depression.' When a patient is organized and able to describe her history and symptom picture so clearly, it can surely be a help to the homeopath.

Sherri was an eager, if a bit nervous patient that first time I saw her ten years ago. She was put together well, with a crisp outfit and recent stylish haircut. She wore quite a bit of make-up, and her nails were freshly manicured and polished.

At twenty five, Sherri worked as a counselor at a local high school and was engaged to be married. She was seeking help for her gynecological issues, concerned about the fact that having HPV infection put her at risk for problems like cervical cancer down the road. (HPV/human papillomavirus is the name of a group of sexually transmitted viruses that can cause genital warts as well as abnormalities in cervical cells—from mild dysplasia to cancer.)

Sherri was also worried about her herpes and the possibility that if she ever became pregnant, a vaginal birth might not be an option because of the risk of passing herpes to the baby. She disliked the antiviral medication she took to treat her herpes; she felt that the treatment was suppressive because she could sense the eruptions just under the surface.

The genital warts she thought she had contracted from a

college boyfriend, though she was not sure. They were small lesions on her labia (which her gynecologist had biopsied), and she experienced no discomfort or other effect from them. She had had irregular Pap test results for several years culminating in the recent procedure to remove the top layer of the cervix. Her fiancé did not have any visible lesions in the genital area.

The herpes simplex she did contract from her fiancé; the first outbreak was two years prior to our visit. The lesion was the size of a quarter on her left labia and quite raw and painful. She had experienced a flu-like feeling and fatigue for weeks before and after the outbreak. Subsequent episodes had been less intense, especially with regard to her systemic symptoms; nonetheless, the lesions were painful and itchy. Sherri could count on getting a herpes lesion before almost every menstrual period. She would also suffer an outbreak if she was under a lot of stress, mostly related to her job.

Sherri felt self-conscious and embarrassed about her health issues; they made her feel 'dirty and gross.' This young woman was very particular about many things, cared a great deal about how others perceived her, and kept her work and home space neat and organized. The worst thing about the HPV and the herpes was that she felt out of control and like she had no say in what her body was doing. She was hoping that homeopathy and other natural medicines might help her, and she was willing to do whatever was suggested.

Sherri had been a high school and college athlete and seemed to take pride in her physical fitness and high energy level. She trained intermittently for mini-triathalons, but often had to forgo training because of her health issues.

In exploring the history of depression Sherri had mentioned on her intake form, I learned that this condition ran in her family, especially on her mother's side. For Sherri, the depression mostly manifested as having very low energy and low self-esteem. She would also feel anxious and worried about almost anything. In recent years, she had felt better emotionally, which she attributed largely to her loving and strong relationship with her fiancé, but she remained concerned that these problems could come back. She suffered a bit from seasonal affective disorder and would always feel at least somewhat better by getting exercise and being outdoors each day.

In the course of our interview, Sherri described the way in which her emotional world was suppressed both in her family and, to some degree, at work. She did not feel she was free to show negative emotions such as anger or frustration. She would just put on a smile and pretend everything was okay. This sort of hiding of emotions took a tremendous amount of energy, and Sherri knew it was not healthy.

A review of Sherri's bodily systems turned up nothing remarkable except for some minor musculoskeletal issues that would arise from sports injuries. She would sweat profusely under her arms when nervous, and she was self-conscious about that. She had numerous warts removed from both her hands and feet; every few years she would have several frozen off. She tended to be on the chilly side and complained of chronically oily skin on her face; she had no problem with acne or other blemishes, just oiliness.

In a case like this, I am always hoping to have a long term impact on the patient. I wanted to see Sherri's Pap test results revert to and stay normal. I wanted to see her have fewer or at least less uncomfortable outbreaks of herpes. I wanted her confidence and self-assuredness to grow. Tall orders for a homeopathic remedy but, in my experience, not unrealistic.

I gave Sherri the remedy *Thuja occidentalis*, one commonly used for issues related to genital warts. Many times, those who need this remedy will have a history of something being suppressed, whether it be a physical complaint or an emotional issue. In Sherri's situation, she spoke about the sense that she was constantly suppressing the herpes with drugs; likewise, at work and within her family, she was always suppressing her emotions. Her additional warts on her hands and feet and the left-sidedness of her herpes were good confirmatory symptoms to indicate *Thuja*. Temperamentally, being overly concerned about what others thought, getting much of her self-definition from her work and from her partner, as opposed to from within, as well as carrying around an underlying feeling of self-disgust—each of these elements also pointed to *Thuja*. Her oily skin and profuse perspiration were additional physical general symptoms indicative of *Thuja*.

I prescribed one dose of *Thuja* 200c and asked to see her two months later. I wanted a few menstrual cycles to go by, to see if we had impacted the herpes. I also wanted Sherri to have results from a follow-up Pap smear. Whenever we can use conventional laboratory results to monitor improvement, we try to do so, in order to provide objective guideposts to judge the efficacy of our treatment.

I also recommended a naturopathic protocol for Sherri's abnormal Pap smears, advising her to stay away from coffee and caffeinated products, alcohol and refined sugars. I also suggested the following supplements:

- Folic acid, 5 mg/day for 3 months only
- Vitamin B-6, 100 mg/day

- Vitamin B-12, 1 mg/day
- Beta-carotene, 50,000 IU/day
- Vitamin C, 1000 mg/day
- Vitamin E, 400 IU/day
- Selenium, 200 mcg/day

This combination of high potency B vitamins and strong antioxidants has been shown to be helpful in such situations. There are other things that can be added or shifted depending on the particular case at hand, but this was the protocol used for Sherri.

When Sherri returned two months later, she came into the office excitedly waving her most recent Pap results: normal. This I would expect based on the procedure she'd had before seeing me; I would want to see at least six months or even a year of normal Pap test results before I would be happy. Based on her previous pathology reports, Sherri was having Pap tests every three months.

Sherri also reported no herpes outbreaks since her last visit, and that she was feeling well and upbeat even though it was the dead of winter when she usually felt emotionally low. Certainly the *Thuja* and the vitamin therapy were helping her. We reduced the folic acid dosage as well as the beta-carotene dosage and kept all else the same. I did not give her any more *Thuja*, but instead decided to wait and see.

At the next follow-up visit, Sherri came in with another good Pap test result and still no sign of the herpes.

Over the course of the last decade, I have continued to see Sherri, and she has done very well. She has had one slightly abnormal Pap test result during these years, which reverted to normal after additional doses of *Thuja*.

I have seen this many times in my practice; women who have had repeated bad Pap test results subjected to procedure after procedure (as they should be) who are quite frightened by such occurrences. When they take the right homeopathic remedy and appropriate supplements, most women I have treated do quite well. Even women who were exposed to diethylstilbestrol (DES) and have more of a potential to have difficulties do surprisingly well.

I always look for overall improvement in the patient, not just a reversal of abnormal Paps or prevention of future abnormal Paps. I look for an improvement in overall energy level, sleep, digestion, and skin, as well as improvement on the mental and emotional levels. I look for an amelioration of other physical troubles—in Sherri's case, for example, the herpes.

Sherri has had herpes outbreaks only a handful of times in the ten years since our initial visit, but has head them off with the use of Lysine, an amino acid which is known to help with the prevention and treatment of herpes. Before I saw her, Sherri had been using Lysine along with her antiviral medication, but without substantial effect; she was still having painful outbreaks at least once a month. Immediately after homeopathic treatment, however, she did not have a herpes outbreak for many months. When she did finally feel one coming on, it was extremely mild and the Lysine did the trick without side effects. This was an immediate and impressive reduction in occurrence, duration and intensity of her herpes outbreaks. While it is true that, over time, many long time herpes sufferers naturally experience a gradual reduction in their outbreaks, with or without any kind of treatment, one would not expect the outbreaks to end so abruptly and become so mild. Yet I have often seen this sort of dramatic response in my herpes patients and find that positive results are the norm for those treated homeopathically and naturopathically.

I have prescribed doses of *Thuja* from time to time for Sherri when her stress is very high or when other acute illnesses arise that are indicative of this remedy. I have also given her the remedy *Lycopodium* at a few junctures when an acute viral illness required it.

Over time and during the course of our many years working together, Sherri has become a confident and self-assured young woman, feeling good both at work and at home. Her mild depression is largely a thing of the past, though she can have low times during the long winters. So, though it is useful in such cases to look at the Pap test results, as always with homeopathy, we look at such results in the context of the whole person.

What I have learned from this and similar cases of HPV and/or genital herpes—some that have responded to *Thuja* and others to different well-prescribed remedies—is that we can help over the long run; the problems might not go away completely, but they can certainly be deeply impacted as the individual patient gets healthier and stronger. At some point, I imagine that Sherri would like to become pregnant and I do wonder how the stress of a pregnancy will impact her system, but I know that she will use me as a resource as needed, based on her happy results with treatment over the last ten years.

Last summer, I ran into Sherri at the start of a local triathlon where my daughter happened to be competing. Looking trim and fit as usual, Sherri was adjusting her water bottle and setting out her biking shoes in the space allowed for the transition between the long swim and the bike ride. I introduced her to my daughter as 'a friend.' Sherri winked at me, looked at my daughter, and said, 'I would never be able to do this kind of event without your mother's help. Good luck in the race!'

Chapter 6

For Older Adults

Getting Older, Getting Better

I will never forget the first time I treated an older patient. I was a mere 26 years old, fresh out of naturopathic medical school, and before me sat a woman of 98 with long, flowing white hair and bright eyes that lit up her face. The fine wrinkles around her mouth broke into an easy smile when I walked into the room. Perhaps she was amused at how young they were letting people practice medicine, and a woman to boot!

She shared her story of deep and overpowering sleepiness ever since she'd had cataract surgery four months earlier. Falling asleep frequently might not seem to be a real complaint in someone of this age, but for this patient, it was. Her 80 year old daughter, who had brought her in to see me, confirmed that her mother had never been like this before the surgery. As I sat in awe of these two older women and the grace, gentleness, and good humor with which they related to one another and the world, I had found yet another reason to love my job.

In 1900, average life expectancy in the US was 47 years. By 2000, that number had increased by about 50 percent to the current age of 74. More than 35 million people, about 12 per cent of the US population, are older than 65. This number will nearly double by 2030. Reports have been published that those born in the early 2000s, many will live to be 100!

The 'very old' (considered to be those older than 85) make up the fastest growing segment of our population at 1.5 per cent. In the year 2000, just 1 out of 5,578 reached the ripe old age of 100; in 2050 that is predicted to rise to 1 out of 472!

Living longer than they used to, people are experiencing more of the effects of aging and general wear and tear than did previous generations. For this reason, health care issues have become central to many of our aging patients. Likewise, adults caring for their own parents must face all manner of health care decisions.

Over the years, I have successfully used homeopathy with older and even with 'very old' patients. I pray that, at 46, I am at the halfway point of my own life. Wouldn't it be nice to live to 92? I envision myself healthy and strong, my mind still clear and my day-to-day life filled with family, friends, work, art and play. Can homeopathy help me and the older people I serve reach a ripe old age? Does using homeopathy along with other preventive measures such as supportive, nourishing, natural medicines offer anything useful to those in their later years? Based on my experience, I certainly believe so, and as the decades fly by, I sure as heck hope so!

For baby boomers entering their 50s and 60s, expectations have shifted considerably from those of the previous generation. Many who come to see me are well informed about their ailments and about natural medicine options. Many have done a decent job of making healthy lifestyle choices in terms of diet, exercise, and the occasional use of botanical medicine or nutritional supplements. They seek homeopathic care for specific concerns, such as digestive disorders, joint problems, cognitive shifts, skin changes, urinary or prostate problems, or issues related to anxiety or depression. Homeopathy is well suited to these patients. We can expect a successful constitutional remedy to improve the chief complaint while also helping the patient's overall well being, energy level, digestion and sleep.

There is no trick to treating the older patient. We homeopaths still take the full case, seeking to understand all elements of the chief complaint and how that fits into the person's overall health. We include a thorough review of the patient's body systems and try to get an understanding of the stresses that impact their lives.

I am also careful to ask about family health history, so that I have a sense of potential genetic predispositions. For instance, if a patient with a strong family history of heart disease comes to see me for something largely unrelated, such as chronic digestive problems or migraines, I will do my best to find a remedy to help that chief complaint; but I will also take time to advise them on topics related to weight loss, proper diet or exercise. A homeopathic remedy can help the migraines, but to counter genetic inheritance, it's important to address lifestyle issues. For patients who find such changes difficult—and many patients of all ages do—I believe that a well-prescribed constitutional remedy will give them a bit more resolve, so they can make the changes they know are necessary.

Sometimes clear-headed older patients without cognitive problems are not so clear about past medical care or the reasons they had particular surgeries or diagnoses. When I first began to practice, this always caught me off guard. How could someone not know why she had a hysterectomy 25 years ago? How could someone not know why their thyroid gland was removed? But it was a different era then; patients were not encouraged to ask questions, and physicians did not always explain.

Even without access to a complete health history, however, there is usually no shortage of information on which to base a homeopathic prescription, so I simply let go of trying to know every detail. As people age, there are usually many examples of imbalance that we can explore, with sufficient colorful detail to all manner of symptoms.

With very old patients, I take more time to understand their living situation and social dynamics. Many experience isolation and loneliness, and I want to understand how that might impact their case. I'm always glad when a relative or support person accompanies them to the appointment, helping to clarify important details of the patient's health history and current complaint. If the patient's main issues are in the mental, cognitive sphere, I'm especially glad to have this support person in the interview to help us. I can take the homeopathic case either way, but it's helpful to have this other voice.

One of my goals when treating older patients is to keep them living independently, if they so choose, functioning well enough to be safe and engaged in life. It is common for older people to have more disability with their illnesses, so while taking the case I also assess this. I try to speak with patients and their family members early on about the sort of care they would like as they age further, or perhaps when they are dying.

I try to be forthcoming and direct without being intrusive, and I hope my patients and their families appreciate this.

Some of my patients in their 70s and 80s have told me that they especially appreciate my taking ample time to hear their stories and trying to understand their situations. In fact, I often feel that I have gained much more than they have from our time together—particularly when a patient has remained optimistic and caring, engaged in life and enthusiastic about something—family, friends, books, nature, community service, music, politics, etc. I am often left inspired and energized by our visits together, and I hope that homeopathy can ease the patient's aches and pains or give them more mental clarity or energy so that they can pursue the things that stir their imagination, spirit, body or mind.

When older patients consult me about a chronic problem, I often find that they have several disease processes occurring at once. For example, I recently saw Jim, a 70 year old man with benign prostatic enlargement who also had frequent bouts of prostatitis, gastro-esophageal reflux (GERD) and seasonal allergies. Multiple diseases like this do not pose a problem for the homeopath, since we prescribe for the whole person. Often we can see patterns in the person's complaints that are helpful to making a prescription.

In Jim's case, for example, he experienced burning pain with each of his complaints: burning in the esophagus, burning on urination, and a burning nasal discharge with his allergies. Seeing such a pattern can lead us to a successful remedy and keep us from being overwhelmed by minutiae. Jim responded very well to the remedy *Arsenicum album*, as do many patients who experience burning sensations with their complaints. Jim's tendency to be very organized, conscientious and anxious when under pressure confirmed the prescription of *Arsenicum*.

I also gave Jim an herbal medicine derived from *Ulmus fulva* (slippery elm) to help coat and soothe the lining of his esophagus. We spoke about some of the basic dietary considerations for those with GERD (not drinking with meals, not lying down after meals, sleeping with an extra pillow, etc.)

At our first follow-up visit two months after taking *Arsenicum*, Jim reported that he was only waking once a night to urinate, down from 3--4 times, and he had not had an episode of prostatitis. As his GERD was markedly improved, he was able to cut out one of his conventional GERD medications.

One thing that always surprises me is the lengthy list of pharmaceutical products many of my older patients are taking. These drugs can produce unwanted side effects—often the very problem the patient is complaining about. The fact that few of these medications are tested in combination during drug studies is of further concern. And we all lack a full understanding of drug and nutrient interactions, which, for many patients who take more than 8 or 10 medications a day, must certainly be a factor. So I spend a fair amount of time with the patient discussing why each medication has been prescribed and in what dosage, how compliant they've been about taking the drug, and whether they experience any known side effects.

The drug history is important to a homeopath because it impacts our understanding of the patient. Am I seeing true symptoms of the patient or symptoms related to the medications they take? Understanding the patient's medications also informs our choice of potency and repetition of the homeopathic medicine. For instance, Gladys, a woman in her 70s, came to see me with end-stage emphysema and lung cancer. She was taking 20 mg of prednisone a day, along with a myriad of other preparations. Rather than give her one dose of a high potency homeopathic remedy as I often do, I gave her the indicated remedy in a 12c potency to take once a day. I felt that the strength and frequency of her other medicines could interfere with the action of the homeopathic remedy if given only once, whereas a lower potency taken more frequently would give the remedy a chance to act. When treating a patient in such a severe condition, I certainly don't expect miracles. I would perhaps expect to gradually (and in conjunction with her other prescribing physicians) reduce Gladys' prednisone level. I would hope to see her become more comfortable and come to some sort of peace with her situation.

Another issue that can arise when treating older patients is their actual ability to take the remedy. Can they open the container and tap out the prescribed number of pellets? If someone is visually impaired or has difficulty using their hands, then I may give a single dose of a remedy in my office.

I am often called upon to treat an older patient who is suffering from an acute illness, be it pneumonia, sinusitis, a urinary tract infection or perhaps issues related to a recent surgery, such as severe constipation or pain at the site of an incision. I love to use homeopathy in such situations because an accurate homeopathic prescription can help the patient avoid taking yet another conventional medication with its probable side effects.

When their general physical symptoms and mental/ emotional symptoms have shifted from their usual constitutional state, these patients may need a true acute remedy. Other times they simply need a dose of their constitutional remedy to help them over a tough spot. I recall the case of one of my older patients, Annabelle, who had come down with pneumonia while in the hospital for a hip replacement. The last thing she needed was all the coughing and difficulty breathing. Her left lower lobe pneumonia, accompanied by severe diarrhea and a high fever, made me think she probably just needed a dose of her constitutional remedy, *Sulphur*. Her daughter administered a dose in the hospital, and Annabelle got over her pneumonia more quickly than her doctors anticipated. She also made a wonderful recovery from the hip surgery.

As to my 98 year old sleepy patient described earlier, she was in a true acute situation, probably a reaction to the anesthesia used during her cataract surgery. The sleepiness, coupled with a dry mouth and a recent, new symptom of constipation, led me to prescribe, for the first time in my then short career, the remedy *Nux moschata*. This brought her back, in short order, to her more robust self. I had the pleasure of treating both mother and daughter for several more years until they passed away, several months apart, when the mother was well past the century mark.

I would like to send this chapter off to my parents, Doris Cynthia Jaffe Rothenberg and Harry Rothenberg, neither of whom made it to the older age, although I imagine they would have really enjoyed those years together. They were both fond of the saying, 'Only the good die young.' How right they were.

The Lovely Man in the Fedora: A Case of Post-Herpetic Neuralgia

During a typical day at work, it's not uncommon for my receptionist to hand me a phone message asking me to call a prospective patient about a specific complaint. The patient or their caregiver usually wants to know if I can help them or their loved one with a particular illness. I will pick up the phone, learn a little about the person with the problem, offer my thoughts, and share bits from my relevant experience.

Such was a phone call I made to 60 year old Richie about post-herpetic neuralgia. This condition, which sometimes follows an outbreak of shingles, can be quite painful and long lasting. Herpes zoster, the medical term for shingles, is caused by the varicella zoster virus, the same virus that leads to chicken pox. Those who have herpes zoster complain of a bubbled rash usually accompanied by pain in a particular skin area related to an underlying nerve—hence the intense neurological pain that sufferers endure. When the rash is present, people may also experience fever and general malaise. Once the rash goes away, the nerve pain usually disappears, too. Sometimes, however, the pain continues long after the rash is gone; this is known as post-herpetic neuralgia and can continue for many months or even years.

Richie's 90 year old father, Frank, was the unlucky patient who had been enduring severe pain for several months, ever since an outbreak of shingles. I told Richie that I'd had good experience treating post-herpetic neuralgia, that the prescription was not routine, and that yes, I would be happy to treat his dad.

Frank arrived a few weeks later with his son and daughter-in-law in tow. He was tall and straight, dressed in a long, grey, cashmere overcoat with a fedora placed squarely on his head. His eyes were a bit rheumy, but his large, strong hands conveyed warmth and sweetness. Here is the story that unfolded.

Frank had had a bout of shingles some three months prior to this visit. The eruption was on his left chest underneath the breast area. It was accompanied by sharp, stabbing sensations, intermixed with a relentless dull ache. His doctors had prescribed antiviral medication and the rash slowly receded. Unfortunately, however, the pain did not; if anything, it seemed to worsen.

What was even more noticeable, especially to his son, was that Frank seemed depressed. Usually quite outgoing and communicative, for the first time in his life Frank preferred to be alone and did not want to be involved with his large, social family. He was losing interest in all the things he had enjoyed into his later years, such as gardening, woodworking, and music.

Like any good homeopathic sleuth, my first question for Frank was, 'What was happening in the months preceding your shingles?' Was there anything in Frank's story or his life that would have made him susceptible to shingles and the ensuing depression, I wondered? Had he become depressed before the shingles outbreak for any reason? This is what I wanted to understand: what *shifted*, so that the course of this healthy, robust person's life had also shifted?

Very occasionally when a homeopath pursues this line of questioning, the patient will answer, 'Nothing happened.' But be persistent! More commonly, perhaps with a bit of prodding, what emerges is a story: an event, experience, realization, trauma or grief that has powerfully impacted the patient. Whether it affected the psyche or the immune system or caused other physiologic reactions, look for what the stressor may have been and how the patient reacted to it. In general, each of us reacts to stressors in patterned and predictable ways. One person may always get a sore throat when under pressure, another a flare-up of a skin condition or digestive problem. The patterned way a person manifests illness is a reflection of their constitutional type. By prescribing that constitutional remedy, we are able to address these underlying tendencies.

It turned out that Frank had had tremendous stress before the shingles outbreak—in fact, several different events had impacted him within a narrow time frame. Sadly, five months before our meeting, Frank had lost his beloved wife of 72 years. His daughter-in-law chimed in to tell me that theirs had been a truly rare relationship of mutual admiration and support. The love that emanated from their household was legendary among their six children and many grandchildren, great-grandchildren, neighbors and friends. How lucky they were to have been blessed with long lives together!

Though Frank seemed to handle his wife's passing with grace and stoicism, one month later he landed in the hospital with a mild heart attack. During the recuperative phase, he developed severe pneumonia and teetered between life and death for several days. After three weeks in the hospital, he finally seemed strong enough to return home. A few days later, the shingles appeared.

When you speak by phone and get only the slimmest sketch of the problem or perhaps just the name of the illness, you can never know the full story of where that diagnosis fits into a particular person's life. This, of course, is the joy and privilege of being a homeopath: understanding people, their lives, and the context for their ailments. How much more compelling to grasp the context and see the person's vital force offering up characteristic symptoms and clear modalities, than simply to treat post-herpetic neuralgia! Unlike our allopathic colleagues who prescribe based on what is *common* about an illness, treating all who have a particular diagnosis in much the same way, we homeopaths work to *understand* the person with the illness and to prescribe individualized treatment based on that person's unique situation.

After hearing many examples of Frank's strength and fortitude, his compassion and need for connection, I knew that his current situation had him veering in another direction. He had reacted to the multiple stressful events in his life with depression, retreat from others, and physical illness—ways that were *atypical* for him. Although I had not treated Frank before, I knew that whatever remedy I would prescribe would be different than what he would have received just a few years back. To me this reflected the idea that he had now moved away from his former constitutional type into a new constitutional state. Because Frank had already been ill for more than three months, I categorized his current condition as a new chronic state —rather than an acute illness.

After the shingles rash disappeared, Frank had been left with the dull ache in his chest interspersed with frequent strong shooting pains. He did not want anything to touch the area. He felt worse with motion, especially of his arms. His only relief was in a hot shower. He was short of breath, a new symptom for him, probably secondary to his serious dance with pneumonia. He was also less steady on his feet. This may not seem unusual for a man in his 90s but it was a big shift for Frank who prided himself on his self-sufficiency and physical abilities.

Since the shingles, Frank complained of a chronic, low-grade headache on the left side; it was nondescript and worse with light. He was struggling with tremendously dry, cracking lips, which might have been due to some of his pain medications. His digestion was good, and his appetite was normal for him with no particular cravings or aversions. He was thirsty for room temperature water. He was generally neither warm nor chilly. He slept on his left side, even with the post-herpetic neuralgia pain there.

He'd been having a serious problem sleeping since this ordeal began and was taking pain medication and sleeping pills; he'd also just begun an anti-depressant. Frank said the pain meds made him sleepy all day, yet he was unable to sleep at night. He was also taking cholesterol and blood pressure lowering drugs.

In my estimation, I had two jobs to do. I needed to help reduce Frank's pain from the post-herpetic neuralgia; but I also needed to address his mounting depression. It could be said, of course, that the chronic pain itself was depressing, but both Frank and his family felt that his depression was more due to feelings of loneliness and sadness about losing his wife and best friend.

In repertorizing Frank's case, I considered symptoms of his pain along with his emotional concerns, and several remedies were strongly represented including *Ranunculus bulbosus*, *Rhus toxicodendron,* and *Natrum muriaticum.* Although the first two remedies covered Frank's physical symptoms well, the *Natrum muriaticum* covered those symptoms *along with* his emotional state—the ill effects of grief, his depression and insomnia, and his preference for being alone. Whenever we are able to address the whole person with one remedy, we should choose that remedy as it will act more deeply and the patient will feel better overall.

I gave Frank one dose of *Natrum muriaticum* 200c and asked him to call in two weeks. I would not want to wait longer than that if the remedy was not correct. I also advised him to talk with his family doctor about discontinuing the antidepressant. He had just begun it, and he didn't like the way it made him feel.

When Frank and his son called back two weeks later, Frank reported that he had no sharp pains in his chest but the dull ache was still there. He reported feeling more energetic and brighter. He had attended a large family gathering and enjoyed the hustle and bustle and being around all the children once again. Frank's son said that his father seemed more himself—interested and engaged in life. I told them this was a good preliminary report and that I would see him in the office two weeks later.

When Frank arrived, I knew right away he was better. He had jauntiness to his gait and a big smile for me. When the subject of his cataracts came up, something we'd not talked about at our first visit, he said, 'Yes, they are definitely an issue, in fact I can hardly see you.' Not missing a beat, I said, 'You know, I'm really very pretty,' to which he quickly replied, 'Oh yes, I know that.' He had a kind of levity and ease and very upbeat energy. That said, he still had the dull ache remaining in his chest; however, his headaches were gone, his lips were healed and his sleep had greatly improved.

At a follow-up visit like this when a patient has done well and the remaining symptoms are covered by the remedy you initially gave, in most cases, you would simply wait or perhaps repeat the remedy. In Frank's case however, several of the things covered by *Natrum muriaticum* were now gone (the mood issues, the headaches, the cracked lips), and they were *completely* gone. I decided that he was no longer in that *Natrum muriaticum* state and that what was left to treat were strictly the local symptoms left by the herpes zoster—a left-sided, post-herpetic, dull ache. The pain was worse when he moved his arms or took a deep breath, and he had itching in the area.

So I decided to prescribe very specifically for his remaining symptoms by giving him *Ranunculus bulbosus* 200c. I had confidence changing remedies this quickly because Frank exhibited a strong vital force, which had reacted well to *Natrum muriaticum* and which presented symptoms clearly. And now, his manifestation of symptoms was clearly pointing to *Ranunculus bulbosus*.

Over the course of several weeks, the dull aches slowly dissipated and Frank felt better than ever. He jumped into projects around the house, and in the several years since I treated him, I hear periodically from his family members that he is doing well.

Post-herpetic neuralgia is a complaint that the conventional medical world is not often able to help. The strong pain medications prescribed may numb or lessen the discomfort, but they come with side effects and other issues. So, do not hesitate to recommend homeopathy in these cases—but be sure to take the whole case and understand the neuralgia in the context of the whole person.

When Frank's son Richie called a few weeks after the *Ranunculus* prescription to give me the preliminary report on his father, he thanked me profusely for my help, saying that he felt like he had his old father back. He wondered if he could ask me an unrelated question. Did I think homeopathy could help his chronic prostatitis?

Chapter 7

Special Topics

Pharmaceuticals, Homeopathy, and Natural Supplements: Can We Use All Together?

When 39 year old Carla first came to see me, she was struggling with anxiety, depression, insomnia, attention deficit disorder, chronic tonsillitis, and fibromyalgia. This single mother of two worked as a computer programmer and was stressed out in all areas of her life— physically, emotionally and financially. She was terribly stiff and sore and had frequent throat infections, but her physical discomforts were overshadowed by her deep anxieties and worries, which were almost paralyzing.

Carla felt chronically overwhelmed at work and at home. She took no pleasure in life and felt there was nothing to look forward to.

For ten years, she'd been receiving medical care for her health complaints but, unfortunately, it didn't seem to be helping much and was costly, too. This just added to her financial burdens while increasing her feelings of despair.

The list of pharmaceuticals that Carla presented to me was impressive. At various times and often in combination she had been prescribed Prozac®, Zoloft® and Celexa® for depression; Ativan®, Valium®, Xanax® and Klonopin® for anxiety; Ambien® and Lunesta® for help with sleep; Adderal® for attention deficit disorder; the anti-inflammatory Celebrex® and the muscle relaxant Flexeril® for fibromyalgia; and a veritable laundry list of antibiotics for her tonsillitis episodes. At the time of our visit, she was on Klonapin®, Celexa®, Ambien® and Adderal®.

Carla is not alone. It is very common for new patients to come to me with a myriad of complaints and a long list of corresponding medications. It used to be mainly my elderly patients, but over the past 20 plus years, increasingly younger and relatively healthier people are coming to me with long lists of drugs they take or have taken. Some of these conventional drugs are amazingly effective or may even be essential for the person's survival. But many others are amazingly ineffective, unnecessary or even detrimental to health. According to a Journal of the American Medical Association article, 108,000 Americans died in 1996 from adverse reactions to FDA-approved medications that had been properly prescribed by licensed medical professionals, and another 2.2 million Americans had negative drug reactions. So, along with the over-prescribing and excessive cost of many drugs, there are growing safety reasons to use caution when beginning new prescriptions or when adding to a drug regimen.

While Carla was frustrated with the conventional medical care she'd received over the past ten years, it was the only kind of care she'd ever had, and she was understandably wary about trying something new. Her main questions to me were: 'Is it worth my time and money to try homeopathy? Can I use homeopathic remedies while still taking my prescription drugs? Can I expect any real results from homeopathy while I'm taking these prescription drugs?'

In my practice, I use homeopathy with almost every patient and have found that it can be used safely alongside or, in some cases, instead of conventional medicines. This makes homeopathy a perfect approach for patients like Carla. I also advise my patients about other things they might do with regard to diet, lifestyle, stress reduction and natural medicine approaches for symptomatic relief as well as prevention of further imbalance and illness. In addition, I help them figure out which prescription and over-the-counter medications they need versus which are more optional and can be safely reduced or stopped.

So, my basic answer to Carla was, yes! Homeopathy can be used to good effect, even when patients are on conventional medications. But the full answer is actually a bit more complicated and, like many things in homeopathy, depends entirely on the individual patient and their story. As for the continuation of Carla's story, we'll get to that a bit later. In the meantime, here are some general thoughts on helping patients who are on conventional medicines to use them judiciously and in conjunction with homeopathic medicines.

As patients begin to feel better from homeopathic treatment, some medications can be safely reduced or discontinued. For instance, antihistamines, decongestants, pain relievers, acne medication or sleep aids, and many drugs used on an 'as needed' basis, can often be decreased or stopped without issue. Even so, I always encourage patients to taper off gradually and in coordination with the prescribing physician; the body does not like change, so the slow and steady route is usually the best way to wean off medication. Some people are impatient, however, and want to throw their medications down the toilet* immediately after beginning care with me; I discourage this. I believe there is a time and place for all sorts of approaches, and being rash (though indicative of certain personalities and corresponding remedy types!) is seldom called for.

Other strong pharmaceuticals such as prednisone, high blood pressure medications, blood thinners, and anti-cholesterol drugs need to be monitored more carefully, and if they can ever be reduced at all, it will only be under strict supervision from the person who prescribed the drug. For example, I have helped numerous patients get off cholesterol drugs like Lipitor®, but we do this slowly, with well-chosen homeopathic remedies and strong changes in lifestyle including diet, exercise and nutritional supplements. It's likely that the homeopathic remedies don't actually lower total cholesterol or triglycerides or raise HDL cholesterol levels as much as support the patient's overall health and give them resolve and focus to make other necessary changes that do shift the blood test values in question. At any rate, the homeopathic remedies work well right alongside the conventional medications.

I have also helped patients reduce their use of powerful steroid medications like prednisone. Because prednisone lessens inflammation, it can be lifesaving and miraculous, but its side effects, especially from long-term use, are very problematic. Prednisone is prescribed for allergic reactions, arthritis, lupus, ulcerative colitis, asthma, psoriasis and many other ailments. Its list of side effects is long and includes increased appetite, restlessness, vertigo, acne, irregular heartbeat, depression, osteoporosis, ulcers, weight gain, changes in body shape from fat redistribution… and the list goes on. It is difficult to stop prednisone when it has been taken for a long time, and any reduction in dosing should always be made under supervision of the prescribing physician.

I have one patient, for example, who had suffered with lupus and was on a high daily dose of prednisone for years before coming to me. With homeopathic treatment as well as stern advice to reduce the stress in her life, her joint pain, muscle aches and depression have decreased greatly, and she has been able to reduce her prednisone from 40 mg to just 5 mg per day and maintain that lower dosage for several years. She does not seem able to get off the drug completely without becoming more symptomatic, but many of the side effects of prednisone are dose dependent, so being on less is a good thing. And over the years, the homeopathic remedies have improved her overall health, even while she remains on the prednisone.

Many patients will need to be on certain medications for life, and no amount of homeopathy or other natural medicine approaches will change that. Replacement-type medicines such as thyroid hormone and insulin are some examples. With homeopathic treatment, however, dosages of these and other drugs may need to be reduced as symptoms, symptom intensity, or blood test values may shift. I often order more frequent lab work to keep an eye on such factors. For example, if I have a patient with adult onset/Type II diabetes who is on the non-insulin drug Metformin® to control blood sugar, and they have been, over many months, able to take well-prescribed homeopathic remedies and commit to dietary changes, consistent exercise and perhaps a small handful of vitamins per day, they may be able to reduce and ultimately get off their Metformin®. But it must be done wisely, with daily blood sugar checks and the support of the prescribing physician.

Sometimes when I'm treating a patient constitutionally that is, for their overall state of health, other acute illnesses arise. For instance, I may be treating someone for arthritis and insomnia when they come down with a bladder infection. I have seen antibiotics antidote constitutional homeopathic care and so I always prefer and have good results treating my patients' acute infections with homeopathy and natural medicines. Like most homeopaths, I really want to see my patients during their acute illnesses because, in addition to helping them through the illness, I get important clues and information about underlying constitutional states and perhaps a view into a remedy they may need in the future.

But if the patient already has begun an antibiotic, either because they could not reach me or they didn't think to use homeopathy for that complaint, I don't go crazy! An occasional antibiotic does not seem to terribly impact a patient. Of course, the repeated use of antibiotics is another story, and we do see negative impacts. Even so, there are times when I believe antibiotics are the very best thing for a patient. If the illness is in any way life threatening or if such infections often lead to worse situations, I will support the antibiotic use and address any adverse results afterward. As far as giving a homeopathic remedy at the same time as an antibiotic, in my experience, it will not hurt, but it will not have a chance to do much either.

So when one of my patients has been on an antibiotic for an infection, I generally ask them to come in a few weeks later to see if we need to re-prescribe a constitutional remedy for their other ongoing chronic complaints.

For people undergoing cancer treatment protocols of chemotherapy or radiation, homeopathic remedies can be used safely to help curb side effects without compromising the desired effect of the cancer treatment. For more, see chapter on Facing Cancer, page 232.

What about birth control pills? I have found that homeopathic remedies can work fine alongside them, but that I may need to repeat a constitutional remedy more often if my patient is taking oral contraceptives. I do have other concerns for my patients who take them, however. For some, I fear that they may risk exposure to sexually transmitted diseases, as they may be less likely to practice safe sex using condoms. For others, the impact of oral contraceptives on the whole body will be extensive, with side effects related to circulation, weight gain, mood changes, etc. And for others, I worry about the effect of long-term use of these pills on fertility. All those concerns aside, homeopathic remedies do work simultaneously for other complaints that women on oral contraceptives may have.

I have also used homeopathy successfully during end-of-life care, even when patients are on strong opiates for pain. The remedies can be a godsend, easing pain on all levels—physical, emotional and spiritual. I also take the opportunity to offer help to care providers when appropriate.

There are really very few instances where homeopathic

remedies cannot be used to good effect alongside conventional medications. But please use care and caution when considering or making changes to your own (or your patient's) medication protocol, and involve the prescribing physicians!

After assuring Carla that she could benefit from homeopathic and natural medical treatment and that, over time, we might even be able to reduce some of her conventional medications, I took her complete medical history. In many ways, her genetic inheritance predisposed her to all of her problems, as her family history was riddled with anxiety, alcoholism, extreme shyness and depression. The external stressors in her life included a deadbeat father of her children, a challenging boss at work and a difficult economy. Carla never felt cared for, and that was the one thing she desperately craved. Her social anxieties and feelings of inferiority, insecurity and self-doubt led to her inability to make decisions and constant dependence on her aging mother for support and encouragement.

Carla's most remarkable physical symptoms included throat infections and tonsillitis three to four times a year. At age 36, she had had her tonsils removed, which was exceedingly traumatic for her; even worse, it had not changed her tendency for sore throats accompanied by very swollen glands. The fibromyalgia, which manifested mostly as wandering joint pain and muscle tension, was worse when she was under more stress, especially at work.

Carla felt like her anxiety caused her attention deficit problems, as she would get so stressed out by demands of her supervisor that her mind would go blank. She would get so overwhelmed with even small tasks at home or related to her children that she would give up, go to her room, and sit on her bed and cry. All this fed back into her feelings of self-doubt, low self-esteem, and insecurity.

After analyzing Carla's case, I chose the remedy *Baryta carbonica* to address both her physical and emotional concerns. This remedy may be indicated for those with a deep feeling of insecurity, indecisiveness, and also immaturity or the inability to take on the responsibilities of adulthood. Carla's tonsillitis and ongoing swollen glands were other symptoms consistent with *Baryta carbonica.* Because of all the medications she was on, I prescribed a daily dose of *Baryta carbonica* in a relatively low potency (12c).

Carla had had many years of conventional treatment without much improvement, so I did not feel she would be at any great risk if she wanted to reduce her medications once she started to feel better from homeopathic treatment. So I asked Carla to speak with her prescribing psychiatrist about the possibility of starting to wean off some of her psychiatric medications if and when she started to improve.

The first thing to go was her Ambien®, which she had been taking 4 or 5 nights a week to help her sleep. As she felt less anxious over the course of several months of homeopathic treatment, she began to sleep better. She would still wake in the night on occasion but was better able to fall back to sleep. At the four month mark and feeling somewhat better with improved sleep and confidence, Carla decided she wanted to try going off the Adderal® for attention deficit issues, which she did, in coordination with her psychiatrist.

On to the Klonapin® for anxiety and Celexa® for depression; but remember, Carla had been on some sort of antidepressant and/or anti-anxiety medication for many years, so I was reluctant to have her stop these anytime soon.

But at a certain point about six months into our work together, Carla announced that she had stopped her Klonapin®. Her therapist, who she saw twice a month, was supportive; he felt like she had been doing better than he'd seen her in years. Her psychiatrist was not thrilled but felt it wouldn't hurt to try—and Carla prevailed.

Since our first meeting, Carla had been on a daily dose of *Baryta carbonica* 12c for two months. As she made gradual improvements and was taking less conventional medication, I moved from daily doses of 12c to single doses of *Baryta carbonica* in the 200c strength, which she'd had twice by the 6 month mark.

At about 18 months into our work together, Carla has greatly reduced her use of conventional drugs. Instead of taking four drugs, she takes only her anti-depressant, Celexa®. She has taken two rounds of antibiotics for throat infections when she was unable to get in touch with me. This was not unusual for her, so we still need to work on her getting fewer infections.

Her fibromyalgia still bothers her but not as much as before, and she uses various natural anti-inflammatory products as needed, such as Curcumin, Bromelain and vitamin C, with some relief. She has begun to date for the first time in many years and has been enjoying her children for the first time, ever. She seems more confident and less needy. She says she doesn't feel as intimidated in social settings and is more willing to take small risks.

Carla has a ways to go in terms of emotional growth, self-confidence, and some of her physical complaints, but over the past 18 months she has evolved into a more self-assured person who is better able to handle the stresses of single motherhood and work. She is grateful for homeopathy and for being able to reduce her conventional medications.

Looking ahead, I do not think Carla will need *Baryta carbonica* for much longer; at a certain point I expect that this remedy will stop helping her as she evolves and her symptoms change. She'll then need a new remedy, but most likely one that is related to *Baryta carbonica*. Perhaps she will need *Pulsatilla* or *Calcarea carbonica*, but I will not be in a rush to change remedies. I will continue to see her every other month or so to keep an eye on her, to answer her questions as they arise, and hopefully to guide her off the Celexa® down the road. By seeing her with some regularity and keeping a pulse on her physical and emotional health, I will be less likely to miss when the next homeopathic remedy is needed.

In my more than two decades of practice, I have often seen patients like Carla who arrive beleaguered from efforts to secure help for their problems. Years and years of drug therapy have given them some help but not enough. From experience, I have come to expect that gentler, more whole-person approaches, especially homeopathy, will often be effective over time. I cannot promise a patient that they will be able to stop all conventional medicines and, in truth, that really is not the goal. The goal is that the person feels better overall, has fewer symptoms, and has more energy to do the things they love.

Can we use homeopathy and other natural medicines at the same time a patient is taking conventional drugs? Absolutely. Do we have to think creatively about homeopathic prescribing and dosing when a patient is already on many medications? Absolutely. Is it worth it? I think so.

Though homeopathy is not a cure-all and has its limitations, we can confidently offer some help for most everyone and a lot of help for some. True, some patients will still be on conventional medications for the rest of their lives, as the benefits outweigh the risks. But patients like Carla show that homeopathy can be a fine tool to help decrease our dependence on pharmaceuticals and help patients find ways to better health.

Too many people on too many drugs does only one thing for certain—it increases the profits of the big pharmaceutical companies! Let's keep working on getting the word out about homeopathy and other natural medicines, for the benefit of our patients, family and friends.

***Note well:** Any unused pharmaceuticals should in fact, not be thrown down the toilet. Small amounts of conventional medications—including hormones, antibiotics, mood stabilizers and many others—have been detected in the drinking water supplies of major metropolitan areas in the US. One way they get there is by people flushing unwanted or unneeded medicines. Another way, which is likely more to blame, is through the body's metabolism of medications and the byproducts that come out in urine and stool. Perhaps this is another reason to reduce dependence on pharmaceutical products, whenever possible.

While there really is no optimal way to dispose of unneeded drugs, experts currently recommend that you place them in a sealed container—along with coffee grounds or kitty litter or something that will make them unusable if found—and place them in the regular trash, to ultimately end up in a landfill.

I Want to Be in the Olympics!

One hot day in 1972, my family sat spellbound around our Magnavox television. Wide-eyed on that cool linoleum floor, we watched Olga Korbut, the spritely Belarusian gymnast, strike a poised position to begin her floor exercise routine. It was the Summer Olympics and this ambassador of goodwill with the remarkable athletic ability was smiling broadly and captivating the crowd. The music began, and I stared enraptured at her muscled physique as she ran fast, then flipped, twirled and danced, performing seemingly impossible feats before ending triumphantly. At that moment, I remember the distinct thought: *I want to be in the Olympics!*

Of course, only a select handful of athletes make it to that elite level. The rest of us, at best, enjoy the friendly competition of a pick-up game of basketball or a swim in the lake, or perhaps we drag ourselves to the gym to get on the treadmill. Although I never realized my childhood vision of becoming an Olympian, little did I know that 36 years later, I would be privileged to work with some high-level athletes who devote most of their waking hours to perfecting their sport. I find it gratifying to use my homeopathy and natural medicine know-how to help these athletes recover from workouts and injuries more quickly, eat optimally, and avoid or get over acute illnesses more effectively. I also enjoy offering support with regard to the mental part of their pursuit, as they strive to reach personal and professional goals.

Interestingly enough, many of these athletes are children. In my own family with three athletes competing at high levels, I've watched them work hard to make breakthroughs and rise to positions of leadership on teams. I've seen them compete with athletes from other backgrounds and cultures, watched differences melt away when the common goals are spelled out, and seen deep friendships forged. I've noticed sports analogies creep into college essays and the lessons taken from athletic pursuits trickle into academic, emotional and spiritual realms. Certainly the positive effects that athletics have on young people are many.

But some young athletes over-train, burn out and set themselves up for lifelong problems with their physical health. They may sustain injuries from lack of appropriate protective gear or from being put in harm's way by overzealous coaches. I have seen kids destroyed by the competition or by being cut from a team. I've seen harsh coaching affect self-esteem and parents push kids to the point of exhaustion. Unfortunately, eating disorders also seem to go hand in hand with certain sports (for example, wrestling, gymnastics, cross country running), and some teachers, trainers, and coaches reinforce unhealthy body images.

Kids at all levels of athletic participation can feel the pressure. Many have been robbed of the fun and spontaneity of outdoor play, pickup games, and finding their own way in sports, as adults have stepped in to organize almost every waking hour of children's lives.

Yet through it all, certain individuals emerge into the world of the elite athlete by a confluence of events: physical ability, access to training and coaching, a particular determination, family support, at least a modicum of luck, and the ability to either sidestep injury or heal completely. In working with these athletes, I have typically found them to be incredibly dedicated to their efforts, single-minded in pursuit of improving their performance, and able to clearly and directly tell me what they need help with. Some come to see me for physical problems, while others ask for help with their mental game or the emotional roller coaster of competing at very high levels. Here are a few of their stories.

An Olympic markswoman in her thirties arrived one day to see me for help with severe migraine headaches. Olivia had come to the sport in her twenties and had quickly risen to the top of her field. But the headaches, which began a few years into her training, were driving her mad. She would lose days at a time to the pain, the nausea, and her utter need to go to bed in a darkened room. Married without children, this sharpshooter was now devoting her entire life to the sport. Her steady arm and sharp eye suited the endeavor. With a high premium on precision, Olivia would commonly hit 99 out of 100 clay shots. And that one she missed would kill her! She was a perfectionist in many aspects of her life but most especially with regard to her training and equipment care. She would not miss a day of shooting and would let nothing interfere with her concentration. She kept her equipment in tip-top shape, and only she herself could prepare her tools of the trade. Her appearance, too, was very tidy, nothing extra or decorative, but rather plain and clean. Her husband, also a marksman, was her only coach, and theirs was an insular and quiet world except for the sound of the rifles! She did wear protective devices for her ears and had had advice about her posture and shooting stance. It was certainly possible that the impact of the recoil coupled with the ear-shattering noise had put her at risk for headaches, but her avocation was not something she would entertain giving up.

Olivia's conscientiousness, her reserved nature, her photophobia which was exacerbated during the headaches, as well as chronic cold sores in and around her mouth all pointed to the remedy *Natrum muriaticum*. Over the course of a year of treatment with this remedy, Olivia's migraines disappeared. Without the distraction of headaches, she has continued to excel in her field. She has since sent me a number of her colleagues for help with various health issues. I have even been invited to try my hand at shooting, but to date have not accepted the offer!

Lydia, a nationally ranked gymnast, came to see me for help with frequent bouts of vertigo. Clearly that sport, really any sport, would not allow for someone to be dizzy! This headstrong and determined 16 year old had already seen many specialists and undergone numerous treatments using conventional medicines and various postural procedures, but to no avail. Each month before her menstrual period, she could count on losing a few days to the vertigo, and she had begun to dread her monthly cycle. The vertigo was wreaking havoc on her competition schedule and her parents, desperate for help, brought Lydia in to see me.

I went about taking Lydia's case, as I do all cases, eventually coming to a broad sweeping review of bodily systems. As it turned out, Lydia also struggled with constipation, likely due to her poor and insufficient diet. Like many gymnasts, dancers, wrestlers and jockeys, she was strongly encouraged to keep an eye on her weight. That, combined with two working parents, late nights at the gym, and sheer fatigue, often meant that her diet suffered.

Lydia had experienced chronic earaches since she was a child and was accustomed to being on antibiotics several times a year. Sometimes the ear infection was discovered by her pediatrician without Lydia having notable symptoms; other times she would have tremendous pain and high fevers. The earaches could be on either side, without discharge. It may be that these chronic earaches had predisposed her to vertigo, but the ear specialist she visited did not think so.

Lydia was a thoughtful, quiet, almost shy girl, who enjoyed her gymnastics team and the other girls in her gym community. She was not as good as some of her teammates, but she kept at it with a kind of dogged determination. It might take her longer to learn certain elements of a routine, but once she had them, she would never forget.

Lydia's general temperament (slower, thoughtful, even plodding) and her physical general symptoms (chilliness, easy perspiration, and tendency for earaches and constipation) led me to the remedy *Calcarea carbonica.* Over the course of three months, Lydia had two doses of *Calcarea carbonica* 200c, which put a stop to her premenstrual vertigo for good. Now back on a full competition schedule, she has been disappointed by her performance this last year, but she vows to keep at it, with her eyes on the 2012 Olympic Summer games.

A major league baseball player in his 30s came to see me primarily for physical complaints but also for help with emotional issues. This strapping utility outfielder, who had been in the big leagues for over a decade, was having trouble with a chronically pulled groin muscle. It had been injured off the field while horsing around with his kids. He had tried anti-inflammatory medications but did not tolerate them well. Although he had followed his trainer's advice for physical therapy and stretching, at the time of our visit, many months after the original injury, he was seemingly no better. It felt worse in the morning and again in the later afternoon. This injury made it difficult for him to hit, field, and run, and he was at his wit's end. He felt that his manager was getting impatient, which made this patient more and more anxious.

The nervousness did not help this man's irritable bowel syndrome. He was chronically gassy and had unpredictable bowels. Being on the road a lot and eating at restaurants did not help. He always traveled with a fiber supplement, which did offer some relief. He also suffered from insomnia related to the anxiety. He worried constantly about losing his spot on the team and letting down his family. When I made a comment about how awesome it was that he had gotten as far as he had, he quickly dismissed it, focusing instead on all he had to lose. He depended greatly on his supportive and loving wife, who traveled with him most of the time with their small children.

I suggested private yoga instruction for him; for those with particular injuries where conscientious efforts at physical therapy have failed, sometimes yoga does the trick. We also discussed dietary changes and ideas for eating on the road that might help to support healthier digestion. I recommended that he stop eating by a certain time each evening, perhaps 7:00 p.m., until the following morning at breakfast, since many with sensitive digestive systems do well with a good 12 hour fast on a daily basis.

Based on this lovely, if self-effacing man's right-sided groin complaint, his digestive difficulties, and his chronic and heightened insecurity, I prescribed the remedy *Lycopodium* over the course of several months. I am happy to say that he experienced steady improvement; his groin area healed completely and his playing got back on track. With his physical complaints on the mend, he was better able to focus on his game and play well; all of which helped his emotional world, too. With less to be stressed about, he was able to enjoy his work and his family. I am sad to say that I have not treated other major league baseball players yet--I hope he will send a few my way!

One of my favorite elite athletes in my practice was Penny, a pint-sized sixth grader and state champion swimmer. Diagnosed with Attention Deficit Hyperactivity Disorder, Penny was almost totally unable to focus in school, and her report card was filled with Ds and Fs. She had frequent angry outbursts, mostly at home, where she would lose her temper, becoming inconsolable and irrational, throwing things, yelling outrageously, screaming, kicking and winding up in a heap of tears. Penny's mother was beside herself trying to help. In fact, each of the four kids in Penny's family seemed to have some major issue that overwhelmed the parents. This caused tremendous stress in the household for Penny and the entire family.

Beyond the swimming, there was little else this diminutive whirlwind had going for her. Sometimes, likely due to the chaotic nature of the household, Penny did not even want to attend a practice or a meet, but as soon as she got there, she was like a single-minded torpedo. Her body was perfect for swimming, and once she stood on the starting block or was in the water, her mind was clear, her goals obvious. Penny had broken records left and right, and was sought after by coaches in the state.

On the physical side, I learned that Penny had chronic loose stools, frequent sinus headaches and recurring fevers (unrelated to the headaches). The fevers came perhaps two or three times a year. She would get very red in the face, glassy-eyed, and droopy, but she had no other symptoms. Her mother had tried treating the fevers with conventional anti-fever meds, but it hadn't seemed to help, so now they waited them out, usually a day or two. Penny had had all manner of lab work to rule out more serious conditions.

Penny's emotional outbursts and inability to control her temper were affecting most aspects of her life, and that is what her mother wanted help with. It was hard to imagine this strong, athletic pixie being difficult, but her mother described some horrific scenarios, way out of proportion to whatever started the situation. For example, a simple, 'No, we cannot go to the store right now,' might ignite World War III.

All that said, when I first met Penny, I fell in love with her. She was bright and spritely with a dazzling twinkle in her eye and an endearing lisp. I never witnessed any of the shenanigans described by her mother, but she and her brothers and sisters were roughing it up in the waiting room the first time I saw her.

I chose the remedy *Belladonna* for Penny because it fit her few physical issues, mostly related to fever and inflammation (that is, red face, glassy eyes, high fever and chronic loose stools). But I also chose it because it fit her behavioral issues. *Belladonna* is on the short list for helping children with poor impulse control, hot tempers that easily flare, and violent outbursts (also consider *Veratrum album, Medorrhinum* and *Nux vomica*). That said, those who need *Belladonna* can be amazingly charming and bright, so that even when they are driving the parent or teacher crazy, they somehow endear themselves to the caregiver at the same time.

In the first year after starting the *Belladonna,* Penny did not have any fevers and her sinus headaches greatly improved. Her stools firmed up to a more typical one time a day. And to her mother's delight, Penny became much calmer at home. A year or so after our first visit, this water wonder finally got into a better school for her, one for children with learning differences. She was not unintelligent, but testing had unearthed a severe auditory processing problem. I believe that with proper teaching geared at the ways she *does* learn, she will continue to improve. She is still an intense kid, and her swimming is still excellent, but she is now much calmer with better control over her impulses. Penny has her eyes on the Olympics in 2012 or 2016, and I hope she makes it! It will be interesting to see if she sustains her interest and dedication to the sport, and can stay healthy, uninjured and motivated with her heavy training schedule.

Although it is a far cry from an athletic field, court or track, sometimes when I am in the clinic all day seeing patients, my work takes on the feeling of an athletic pursuit. Listening to patients' stories one after another for many hours requires endurance. Like an athlete, I need to be comfortable in my own body, undistracted by the surroundings; I need to be 'in the zone.' For a physician, this means knowing the rudiments of case taking. It's equivalent to being able to dribble a basketball without looking, a skill practiced over time to make it seamlessly second nature. It means being open, using all the senses to observe/perceive the patient, just as an athlete develops court or field sense, and instantly reacts with small and large adjustments to the case-taking strategy. It means basing clinical decisions on hard-earned study, practice and experience, informed by the current environment and patient, and aiming for a successful outcome all the way around.

When I am in the zone at the clinic, the hours spin right off the clock and the day zips by. Asking the right question at the right time — which may seem easy to preceptors sitting in or students watching a case being taken—actually is an outgrowth of honed perception skills and being acutely attuned to the patient before you. Asking those correct questions allows the case to unfold easily and the patient to receive a helpful remedy. Like an athlete, I put a lot of effort into getting into the zone with patients and creating ways to have predictable and easy access to it, day in day out. For every practitioner finding that place and keeping easy channels to it will be done in different ways. For me, it stems from the ability to quiet my mind, to close out other distracting thoughts or needs. I do that by taking responsibility for being well rested, well exercised and well fed! I make lists in the morning, that I add to during the day, of things I need to accomplish or take care of, so I don't worry I will forget the minutiae that make up being a doctor, mother, wife, community member, etc. I also keep close to the surface of my mind that this patient, whichever patient it is, has come to me for help. They are suffering in some way, and it is my job to try my hardest, without distraction, to help them. It is really my only job at that moment; I put a high premium on being focused. I can pull my personal resources together to that moment in time and place, for the purpose of understanding and supporting my patient. In ways, this process for me is very liberating as it's my *only* job at that moment, and though I 'muti-task' in the case taking itself — by being observant, letting my observations inform my questions, being aware of interactions within the room, etc., it is still *much* easier than say running a household with three teenagers! So, part of what I do in my teaching other homeopaths is to just bring these ideas out into the open. By just mentioning it, I can help other providers start thinking about their own skills and strengths in this regard and help future providers be better able to help their patients.

Perhaps the single most important element for an athlete to excel among other successful athletes is a tough mental game enabling them to get *and* stay in the zone,' to get over losses quickly, to take feedback, to integrate that advice with grace and to stay focused regardless of what the surrounding environment might throw their way (for example weather, court conditions, equipment issues, the crowd, judges and referees). There are many books to help athletes work on their inner or mind game. A few of my current favorites, highly recommended by my son, Jonah are: *Mind Gym, An Athlete's Guide to Inner Excellence* by Gary Mack and David Casstevens, *The Inner Game of Tennis: The Classic Guide to the Mental Side of Peak Performance* by Timothy Gallwey, *Sacred Hoops* by Phil Jackson, and *The Way of the Peaceful Warrior* by Dan Millman.

I rarely see a serious athlete for homeopathic treatment without also broaching the subject of other natural medicine approaches. For example, I frequently work with them to optimize their nutrition by creating an appropriate, individualized diet and supplement regimen. Elite athletes and privately coached individuals often have already had nutritional advice from other professionals, but a surprising number of athletes have not. Many athletes overlook the need for healthy protein to build and maintain strong muscles.

Especially those who are vegetarian or vegan, I will review good sources of easy-to-have-on hand sources of protein that are not all soy-based such as nuts and other legumes such as garbanzo and kidney beans.

I am also happy to recommend natural medicine protocols to prevent injuries, decrease lactic acid build-up after strenuous exercise, and promote healing, especially after a big event. Bromelain, the enzyme derived from pineapple, along with vitamin C should be in every athlete's gym bag. Both will help to reduce inflammation and adhesion formation and act as gentle anti-inflammatory agents to help with tissue repair. I refer to massage therapists, cranial osteopaths, yoga teachers, chiropractors, and other physicians. If an athlete seems open, I may suggest psychological work such as mindfulness meditation or sports psychology therapy or recommend particular books (see above).

Staying healthy before and during competitions, especially when athletes are on the road, is another important concern. For example, if there is a tendency for constipation, I recommend bringing along a fiber supplement. If the water supply is not known to be reliable, beyond recommending bottled water, I suggest acidophilus to help build healthy flora in the gut. I have many of my traveling patients bring along charcoal tablets (not capsules). These can be put to good use for a sore throat, for traveler's diarrhea, or crushed up and put on a bug bite. Taken orally, charcoal will turn the stool black and can interfere with some medication like the birth control pill, so users beware! But the short term use is effective and benign; it is inexpensive, stays potent in all weather, and does not go bad over time.

I love working with athletes, as they are determined, disciplined and compliant, wanting to optimize their performance. That said, high-level athletics do put a strain on the patient's physical, mental and emotional worlds. Stressors, even the good ones, cause patients to develop symptoms in reaction to the stress. And those symptoms tend to arise in predictable and patterned ways, depending largely on the constitutional type of the person. That's where homeopathy comes in! Treat the whole person, support the body's inborn abilities to strike balance and find health, and you will help the athletes in your life or practice immeasurably.

The world of sports and athletics offers so much physically, psychologically, emotionally and even spiritually. We providers of natural medicine should do whatever we can to help athletes optimize performance, reduce the chance of injury, heal injuries that occur, and add to the positive mental game. Homeopathy–with its safe, effective remedies that will not turn up on a drug test–is the perfect thing to offer elite athletes. As I say to my now grown kids, each elite athletes in their own right: Play hard, play fair!

In Conclusion

Over the years that I have written these pieces the entire posture toward complementary and alternative medicine has shifted. Openness on the part of the medical world, demand from patients and scientific research continue to grow these natural medicine approaches. It is my hope that in the coming decades the best medicine will be the medicine that is most appropriate to each patient at the times they are ill. I dream that a perfect integration of orthodox and natural medicine approaches will be the norm and the expectation. Patients whole stories will be taken into account and a wide range of approaches will be entertained. I also hope that in the US a health care plan will cover all of our citizens, not just those who can afford it and that the true value of CAM medicine will be realized for all. So, a few short words of final advice: eat well, try to exercise regularly, find outlets for the big stressors in your life, create healthy and mutually supportive relationships and get enough sleep! Be well!